FASTtrack

Applied Pharmaceutical Practice

Christopher A Langley
Senior Lecturer in Pharmacy Practice,
Aston University School of Pharmacy,
Birmingham, UK

and

Dawn Belcher
Teaching Fellow, Pharmacy Practice,
Aston University School of Pharmacy,
Birmingham, UK

Pharmaceutical Press
London • Chicago

Published by the Pharmaceutical Press
An imprint of RPS Publishing
1 Lambeth High Street, London SE1 7JN, UK
100 South Atkinson Road, Suite 200, Grayslake, IL 60030-7820, USA

© Pharmaceutical Press 2009

(**PP**) is a trade mark of RPS Publishing
RPS Publishing is the publishing organisation of the Royal Pharmaceutical
Society of Great Britain

First published 2009

Typeset by J&L Composition Ltd, Scarborough, North Yorkshire
Printed in Great Britain by TJ International, Padstow, Cornwall

ISBN 978 0 85369 835 7

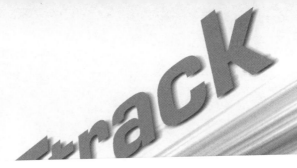

Books are to be returned on or before
the last date below.

al

Contents

Introduction to the *FASTtrack* series

FASTtrack is a new series of revision guides created for undergraduate pharmacy students. The books are intended for use together with textbooks and reference books as an aid to revision to help guide students through their exams. They provide essential information required in each particular subject area. The books are also useful for pre-registration trainees preparing for the Royal Pharmaceutical Society of Great Britain's (RPSGB's) registration examination, and for practising pharmacists as a quick reference text.

The content of each title focuses on what pharmacy students really need to know in order to pass exams. Features include*:
- concise bulleted information
- key points
- tips for the student
- multiple choice questions (MCQs) and worked examples
- case studies
- simple diagrams.

The titles in the FASTtrack series reflect the full spectrum of modules for the undergraduate pharmacy degree.

Titles include:
Complementary and Alternative Medicine
Managing Symptoms in the Pharmacy
Pharmaceutical Compounding and Dispensing
Pharmaceutics: Dosage form and design
Pharmaceutics: Drug delivery and targeting
Pharmacology
Physical Pharmacy (based on Florence and Attwood's Physicochemical Principles of Pharmacy)
Therapeutics

There is also an accompanying website that includes extra MCQs, further title information and sample content: www.fasttrackpharmacy.com.

If you have any feedback regarding this series, please contact us at feedback@fasttrackpharmacy.com.

*Note: not all features are in every title in the series.

Preface

This book has been written as a supplement to *Applied Pharmaceutical Practice* (Langley and Belcher, 2008) to further guide the student pharmacist or pharmacy technician through the main stages involved in pharmaceutical dispensing and to provide a number of exercises for self-assessment. The aim of this book is to provide students with an additional reference text to accompany the compulsory dispensing courses found in all undergraduate MPharm programmes and equivalent technical training courses.

Christopher A Langley
Dawn Belcher
Birmingham, UK
January 2009

About the authors

Christopher A Langley, BSc, PhD, MRPharmS, MRSC, FHEA

Chris Langley is a qualified pharmacist who graduated from Aston University in 1996 and then undertook his pre-registration training at St Peter's Hospital in Chertsey. Upon registration, he returned to Aston University to undertake a PhD within the Medicinal Chemistry Research Group before moving over full time to pharmacy practice. He is currently employed as a Senior Lecturer in Pharmacy Practice, specialising in teaching the professional and legal aspects of the degree programme.

His research interests predominantly surround pharmacy education but he is also involved in research examining the role of the pharmacist within both primary and secondary care. This includes examining the pharmacists' role in public health and the reasons behind and possible solutions to the generation of waste medication.

Dawn Belcher, BPharm, MRPharmS, FHEA

Dawn Belcher is a qualified pharmacist who graduated from the Welsh School of Pharmacy in 1977 and then undertook her pre-registration training with Boots the Chemist at their Wolverhampton store. After registration she worked as a relief manager and later as a pharmacy manager for Boots the Chemist until 1984. While raising a family she undertook locum duties for Boots the Chemist and in 1986 became an independent locum working for a small chain of pharmacies in the West Midlands while also working for Lloyds Chemist.

In 1989 she began sessional teaching with the Pharmacy Practice group at Aston University which continued until she took a permanent post in 2001. She now enjoys teaching practical aspects of pharmacy practice while still keeping an association with Lloydspharmacy where she is employed as a relief manager.

Abbreviations

ACBS	Advisory Committee on Borderline Substances
ACE	angiotensin-converting enzyme
ADHD	attention deficit hyperactivity disorder
CD	controlled drug
CDA	completely denatured alcohol
CHI	community health index
CHIP	Chemicals (Hazard Information and Packaging for Supply) Regulations
CMP	clinical management plan
Defra	Department for Environment, Food and Rural Affairs
DPF	*Dental Practitioners' Formulary*
ESPS	essential small pharmacies scheme
ETP	electronic transmission of prescriptions
FHSAA	Family Health Services Appeal Authority
GDC	General Dental Council
GMC	General Medical Council
GOC	General Optical Council
GP	general practitioner
GSL	general sale list
HIV	human immunodeficiency virus
HPC	Health Professions Council
HRT	hormone replacement therapy
HSW	Health Solutions Wales
ID	identification
IDA	industrial denatured alcohol
IMS	industrial methylated spirit
MAOIs	monoamine oxidase inhibitors
MDI	metered dose inhaler
MHRA	Medicines and Healthcare products Regulatory Agency
MMS	mineralised methylated spirits
MURs	medicines use reviews
NCSO	no cheaper stock obtainable
NHS	National Health Service
NHSBSA	National Health Service Business Services Authority
NMC	Nursing and Midwifery Council
OP	original pack
OTC	over the counter
P	pharmacy medicine
PCO	primary care organisation
PCT	primary care trust

PGDs	patient group directions
PIL	patient information leaflet
PIN	personal identification number
PMR	patient medication record
PO	pharmacy only
PODs	patients' own drugs
POM	prescription-only medicine
PPD	Prescription Pricing Division
PSD	Practitioner Services Division
RPSGB	Royal Pharmaceutical Society of Great Britain
SLS	selective list scheme
SOP	standard operating procedure
SPC	summary of product characteristics
TSDA	trade-specific denatured alcohol
TTA	to take away
TTO	to take out

chapter 1
Introduction, medicines classification and standard operating procedures

Overview

Upon completion of this chapter, you should be able to:
- understand the layout of this book and the broad contents of the different chapters
- describe the different categories of medicines classification
- be able to use standard operating procedures (SOPs) and understand the role that they play within pharmacy.

Introduction and overview

Layout of this text

The supply of medicines is a basic function of pharmacists and pharmacy technicians. With the advent of clinical pharmacy and the introduction of 'new roles' for pharmacists, the content of pharmaceutical education has altered to reflect these additions. However, the supply of medicines remains a key component of the role of pharmacy within modern healthcare and, therefore, it is vital that all pharmacists and pharmacy technicians are competent in medicines supply.

This text has been designed to guide the student pharmacist or pharmacy technician through the main stages involved in safe and effective medicines supply. The aim of the book is to provide student pharmacists with an additional supporting revision text to accompany the compulsory dispensing courses found in all MPharm programmes and to reinforce the concepts discussed in *Applied Pharmaceutical Practice* (Langley and Belcher, 2008). In addition, it will be of equal value for student pharmacy technicians during their educational courses.

Chapters 1–10 are set out as follows:
1. A **chapter overview** box summarising the main points contained within the chapter.
2. An **introduction and overview** of the key material covered within the chapter.

3. Where appropriate, a collection of **worked examples** (Chapters 1–7) to further aid understanding and to include details on suitable labelling and packaging.

4. A series of **self-assessment questions** which it is expected that the student would work through independently. The answers to the questions can be found at the end of the book (in Chapter 11).

KeyPoint

To gain the most from this text, it is suggested that the reader has access to either the print or online version of a recent copy of both the *British National Formulary* and the respective *Drug Tariff* for their country (England and Wales, Northern Ireland or Scotland).

To guide the reader through the different topics relating to medicines supply, this book has been divided into a number of different chapters, which reflect the chapters of the parent volume (*Applied Pharmaceutical Practice*) and are as follows.

Chapter 1 Introduction, medicinal classification and SOPs

Chapter 1 introduces the text and provides an outline of the key points behind medicines supply. It also covers the basic classification of medicines and the role of standard operating procedures.

Chapter 2 NHS supply in the community 1: prescription forms and prescribing

Chapter 2 provides an overview of medicines supply in the community. NHS prescription forms and the restrictions placed on different NHS prescribers in the community, including the role of the UK *Drug Tariffs*, are covered.

Chapter 3 NHS supply in the community 2: prescribers and the dispensing process

Chapter 3 discusses the different NHS prescribers within the community. Following on from this is an overview of the dispensing process which should be followed when supplying medicines against NHS prescription forms, along with a collection of worked examples.

Chapter 4 NHS supply within hospitals

Chapter 4 covers the supply of medicines via the NHS within hospitals.

Chapter 5 Non-NHS supply

Chapter 5 contains similar material to Chapters 2 and 3, focusing on non-NHS supply, including the supply of medication against private prescription forms and via oral and written requisitions.

Chapter 6 Controlled drugs

Chapter 6 uses some of the material already discussed in Chapters 2–5 and summarises the laws and regulations relating to the supply of controlled drugs, via both NHS and non-NHS routes.

Chapter 7 Emergency supply

Chapter 7 reinforces the key points behind the emergency supply of medicines by a pharmacist, at the request of both a prescriber and a patient.

Chapter 8 Patient counselling and communication 1: the basics of patient communication

Chapter 8 provides an overview of the basics of patient communication ensuring that pharmacists and pharmacy technicians are familiar with both verbal and non-verbal communication, and able to communicate effectively with patients and carers.

Chapter 9 Patient counselling and communication 2: product-specific counselling points

Chapter 9 summarises important counselling points that need to be considered for specific dosage forms, and is a useful reference source to enable students to answer parts of the self-assessment questions from other chapters.

Chapter 10 Poisons and spirits

This chapter discusses the key points behind the supply of poisons and spirits from pharmacies.

Chapter 11 Answers to exercises

The final chapter contains answers to the exercises found in earlier chapters of the book.

Medicines classification

The Medicines Act 1968 defines three classes of medicinal products for human use: general sale list (GSL) medicines, pharmacy (P) medicines and prescription-only medicines (POM).

KeyPoints

This revision text has been designed to provide student pharmacists and technicians with a supporting revision text to accompany the compulsory dispensing courses found in all MPharm and technician education programmes.

To gain the most from this book, we suggest using the examples contained within it alongside the parent volume, *Applied Pharmaceutical Practice* (Langley and Belcher, 2008), which goes into more detail about the topics summarised in the chapters in this text.

KeyPoints

The Medicines Act 1968 defines three classes of medicinal products for human use:

- general sale list (GSL) medicines
- pharmacy (P) medicines
- prescription-only medicines (POMs).

General sale list medicines

These are medicines that can be purchased from a wide range of shops, general stores, supermarkets, newsagents, petrol stations, etc. Products classified as GSL are considered to be reasonably safe and therefore can be sold without the supervision of a pharmacist.

Products categorised as GSL medicines have strict controls concerning their strength, use, pharmaceutical form and route of administration. The maximum dose or maximum daily dose is also controlled for medicines for internal use. Another control that may be enforced is pack size with a limit to the size of pack allowed as a GSL medicine.

The following classes of medicinal products for human use are not allowed to be classified as GSL medicines:

- enemas
- eye drops
- eye ointments
- products containing aspirin or aloxiprin and intended for administration either wholly or mainly to children
- products for parenteral administration (a product given by injection, bypassing the enteral (gastrointestinal) tract)
- products used as anthelmintics (a substance that expels or destroys intestinal worms)
- products used for irrigation of wounds, the bladder, vagina or rectum.

Pharmacy medicines can be sold only from a pharmacy under the supervision of a pharmacist. It should be noted that, although the sale of GSL medicines from a pharmacy does not need to be under the supervision of a pharmacist, GSL medicines must still be sold under the 'personal control' of a pharmacist.

The term 'personal control' comes from the Medicines Act 1968 and has never been interpreted in the courts. However, it is generally understood to mean that the pharmacist must be available on the premises. If a pharmacist is not available, no medicines (including GSL items) may be sold at all. For this reason, GSL medicines sold from pharmacies are often treated as P medicines. Obviously, this restriction does not apply to GSL medicines sold from other (non-pharmacy) establishments.

KeyPoints

General sale list **(GSL)** medicines are medicines that can be purchased from a wide range of shops, general stores, supermarkets, newsagents, petrol stations, etc.
Products classified as GSL are considered to be reasonably safe and therefore can be sold without the supervision of a pharmacist.

Pharmacy medicines

These may be sold from pharmacies under the supervision of a pharmacist. The pharmacist or the pharmacy technician/counter assistant asks a number of questions before making the sale to ensure that the medication is safe for the patient and advice as to the use of the product is provided. Some medicines may be sold only when certain criteria have been met, e.g. when supplying emergency hormonal contraception from a community pharmacy.

A P medicine is the definition given to medicinal products not included on the prescription-only medicines order or the general sale list or is a product that is supplied outside the GSL package limit or maximum dosage limit. A few medicines are called pharmacy-only (PO) medicines and include medicines that would normally be included on the GSL list but where the manufacturer has limited the supply of the medicines to pharmacies only.

> **KeyPoint**
>
> **Pharmacy (P)** medicines may be sold from pharmacies under the supervision of a pharmacist.

Prescription-only medicines

These medicines are usually obtained on the authorisation of a valid prescription form (either an NHS or a private prescription form), written by a recognised prescriber registered in the UK and presented at a registered pharmacy (although exceptions to this do exist, e.g. dispensing doctors, inpatient hospital supply and emergency supply at the request of a patient).

Traditionally the prescriber would have been a doctor or a dentist but, with recent changes to healthcare legislation and the introduction of supplementary and independent prescribers, the term 'prescriber' includes many other healthcare professionals such as suitably qualified nurses and pharmacists.

Medicines may also be exempted from POM classification if there are limitations on the use of the product. An example would be hydrocortisone cream 1% normally categorised as POM, but a P medicine in packaging that limits the use of the cream to the treatment of allergic contact dermatitis, irritant dermatitis, insect bite reactions and mild-to-moderate eczema; it should be applied sparingly once or twice a day for a maximum of 1 week. The P or 'over-the-counter' (OTC) form is licensed only for those indications and dosages, and further restriction to sales include unsuitability for OTC sale to treat:

- children under 10 years
- conditions on the face or anogenital area

> **KeyPoints**
>
> **Prescription-only medicines (POMs)** are medicines that are described in the Prescription Only Medicines (Human Use) Order 1997. They are usually obtained on the authorisation of a valid prescription form (either an NHS or a private prescription form) written by a recognised prescriber registered in the UK, presented at a registered pharmacy (although there are exceptions).
>
> Traditionally the prescriber would have been a doctor or a dentist but, with recent changes to healthcare legislation and the introduction of supplementary and independent prescribers, the term 'prescriber' includes many other healthcare professionals such as suitably qualified nurses and pharmacists.

- conditions where the skin is broken or infected including cold sores, acne and athlete's foot
- pregnant women.

Medicines containing controlled drugs are generally given a POM classification. Exemptions to this general rule include where the strength of the controlled drug included in the medication is below a certain value and when the medicine ingredient is covered by Schedule 5 of the Misuse of Drugs Regulations 2001.

Standard operating procedures

KeyPoint

Standard operating procedures are often referred to as 'SOPs' and include all the written protocols and procedures in place within a pharmacy.

Standard operating procedures are often referred to as 'SOPs' and include all the written protocols and procedures in place within a pharmacy. They state the way that the pharmacy expects tasks to be carried out to ensure provision of a quality service. They include, for example, the questions that must be asked of a patient so that his or her needs can be correctly identified and appropriate action taken.

The history of SOPs

Standard operating procedures, in their current form, have existed for the dispensing supply process since January 2005. They were put in place to ensure clinical governance of the dispensing procedure. 'Clinical governance' is the term used in the National Health Service (NHS) and private healthcare system to describe a systematic approach to maintaining and improving the quality of patient care.

As pharmacies differ so much, a single SOP could not be devised that would cover all pharmacies. Therefore each pharmacy has individually tailored SOPs for their working environment. Larger companies, with numerous pharmacies, may have single SOPs that cover all their premises. These were formerly known as *company policy*. It is considered good practice to have SOPs in place for all procedures carried out in the pharmacy.

What are the advantages of SOPs?

1. They can assist with quality assurance, ensuring that patients receive a service that meets certain predefined standards.
2. They ensure consistency, which helps to maintain the level of service offered and therefore maintain good pharmaceutical practice at all times.
3. They help 'free time' for pharmacists, by enabling the delegation of certain tasks. This in turn enables pharmacists to engage in some of the 'new roles' and provides enhanced

roles for pharmacy technicians that recognise their specific
expertise.
4. They set out clear lines of accountability, ensuring that staff
   are aware of their own responsibilities.
5. They help locum and part-time staff understand the processes
   and running of the pharmacy.
6. They are useful templates in the training of new staff.
7. They provide additional information for the audit process.

The preparation of SOPs

The Royal Pharmaceutical Society of Great Britain (RPSGB)
breaks down the preparation of an SOP into six stages:
1. **Objectives:** the purpose of the SOP.
2. **Scope:** what are the areas of work to be covered by the SOP?
   It is advisable that this should not be over-complex.
3. **The stages of the process:** this is a description of how the task
   is carried out. It is important that this description is clear and
   unambiguous, preferably without the use of jargon.
4. **Responsibility:** who is responsible for carrying out the
   procedure and who ensures that staff members are suitably
   trained to carry out a procedure? In a working pharmacy this
   would also include contingency plans detailing what to do in
   cases of sickness or holiday leave, etc.
5. **Other useful information:** for example, details on how the
   SOP is to be audited. Auditing the processes helps maintain
   standards and identifies any areas where improvement could
   be made.
6. **Review:** shows how the process is monitored to ensure that it
   remains up to date and relevant.

The new pharmacy contract for England and Wales

The new pharmacy contract (since April 2005) divides the
activities that community pharmacies undertake into three tiers
of service: essential services, advanced services and enhanced
services. The essential services provided by a community
pharmacy are compulsory and the minimum required of a
contractor as part of the pharmacy contract.
   There are seven essential services identified in the contract:
1. Dispensing
2. Repeat dispensing
3. Disposal of unwanted medicines
4. Promotion of healthy lifestyles (public health)
5. Signposting (provision of information on where and how to
   access other healthcare and social care providers)
6. Support for self-care (help to minimise the inappropriate use
   of healthcare and social care services)
7. Clinical governance.

A similar contract exists within Scotland, with four core services: an acute medication service (AMS), a minor ailment service (MAS), a chronic medication service (CMS) and a public health service (PHS). Additional services are to be agreed locally but on the basis of national (Scottish) specifications.

A pharmacy must have in place SOPs for all these activities. In addition other SOPs are developed to aid the business, e.g. an SOP covering OTC sales (sale of medicines and provision of advice), stock ordering and receipt of goods (ensuring that stock received is what was ordered, is in date and does not have a short shelf-life, and is to be stored correctly) and the receipt of telephone calls, should be in place.

Worked examples

Example 1.1
An SOP for the reception of a prescription form within a community pharmacy

A summary of how to dispense NHS and non-NHS prescriptions can be found in the subsequent chapters of this book. However,

Figure 1.1 An example of a standard operating procedure for the reception of a prescription form within a community pharmacy.

STANDARD OPERATING PROCEDURE – DISPENSING	
PRESCRIPTION FORM RECEPTION (NHS)	
OBJECTIVES	To maintain good patient relations To ensure that the prescription form presented relates to the named patient To ensure safe dispensing To ensure that details on the reverse of a prescription form are correctly filled out, and any applicable fee is collected To ensure effective communication between patient and pharmacist
SCOPE	The reception of all NHS prescription forms brought into the pharmacy by patients or their representatives Prescription forms received in bulk (prescription form collection service) or those received by telephone call are excluded from this SOP
STAGES OF THE PROCESS	Greet patient in friendly manner Check name and address of the patient (rewriting it if handwritten and unclear) Check that the reverse of the prescription form is filled out correctly If the prescription form is for a child, check the age or date of birth is specified Collect any prescription charge(s) and indicate this on the prescription form Indicate whether or not the patient or patient's representative is waiting or calling back and whether or not the patient or patient's representative has requested to see the pharmacist Pass the prescription form through to the dispensary for prompt processing
RESPONSIBILITY	All staff members working on the medicines counter
OTHER USEFUL INFORMATION	Audit carried out by pharmacist (or designated technician/supervisor) using the basic objectives and the stages of the process as a basis of the audit
REVIEW	Following audit, make time to review findings with all staff so that any deficiencies can be rectified and any points of good practice can be implemented within the whole group, not just on an individual basis

consider an SOP for the dispensing of prescriptions (i.e. service number 1 from the list of essential services above). This can be broken down into a number of stages:

1. Prescription reception
2. Professional check
3. Intervention and problem solving
4. Label generation and collection of prescription item(s)
5. Accuracy checking
6. Handing out prescription item(s) to patients or their representatives
7. Dealing with 'owings' when prescription forms are incompletely filled.

The list above covers the basic dispensing procedure and each stage requires an SOP. Figure 1.1 contains an example of an SOP for the reception of a prescription form within a community pharmacy.

Figure 1.2 An example of an audit form for the audit of a standard operating procedure for the reception of a prescription form within a community pharmacy.

STANDARD OPERATING PROCEDURE – DISPENSING
PRESCRIPTION FORM RECEPTION (NHS) – Audit

NAME OF AUDITOR: _____ DATE OF AUDIT: _____

| AUDIT QUESTION | SATISFACTORY | | AREAS OF NON-COMPLIANCE | RECOMMENDATIONS |
	YES	NO		
1. Are patients/representatives greeted in a friendly manner?				
2. Is the identity of the patient checked (i.e. name and address)?				
3. Is the reverse side of the prescription form checked for signatures and completion?				
4. Is any applicable fee collected and noted on the prescription form?				
5. If the prescription form is for a child, is the age or date of birth checked?				
6. Is information transferred between patient and pharmacist (call back, waiting, request for advice)?				
7. Are prescription forms promptly passed to the dispensary?				

REVIEW DATE: _____ REVIEWED BY: _____

Example 1.2
An audit form for the audit of an SOP for the reception of a prescription form within a community pharmacy

In order to ensure that each SOP is being followed properly and that it is functioning correctly, periodic audits of the processes covered by SOPs are carried out. Figure 1.2 contains an example of an audit form for the audit of an SOP for the reception of a prescription form within a community pharmacy.

Further examples of SOPs can be found in *Applied Pharmaceutical Practice* (Langley and Belcher, 2008).

Self-assessment

For questions 1–7 below, **ONE** or **MORE** of the responses/statements is/are correct. Decide which of the responses/statements is/are correct and then choose:

A   If statements 1, 2 and 3 are all correct.
B   If statements 1 and 2 are correct and statement 3 is incorrect.
C   If statements 2 and 3 are correct and statement 1 is incorrect.
D   If statement 1 is correct and statements 2 and 3 are incorrect.
E   If statement 3 is correct and statements 1 and 2 are incorrect.

Question 1
1. **POMs cannot be sold to members of the general public.**
2. **PO medicines are GSL medicines where the manufacturer has limited the supply of the medicines to pharmacies only.**
3. **P medicines are any medicinal products not included in the Medicines (Products other than Veterinary Drugs) (General Sale List) Order 1984 or the Prescription Only Medicines (Human Use) Order 1997.**

Question 2
1. **In pharmacies all GSL medicines must be sold under the supervision of a pharmacist as defined by the Medicines Act 1968.**
2. **In pharmacies all PO medicines must be sold under the supervision of a pharmacist as defined by the Medicines Act 1968.**
3. **In pharmacies all GSL medicines must be sold under the personal control of a pharmacist as defined by the Medicines Act 1968.**

Question 3
With the exception of some controlled drugs, when prescribing a medical practitioner may do the following:
1. **Prescribe any GSL medicine within its product licence.**

2. Prescribe any P medicine within its product licence.
3. Prescribe any POM medicine within its product licence.

Question 4
Which of the following are classes of medicinal products for
human use as defined by the Medicines Act 1968?
1. POM – prescription-only medicine
2. GSL – general sale list medicine
3. PO – pharmacy-only medicine

Question 5
Which of the following types of medicinal product for human use
CANNOT be included in the general sale list (GSL) even though
the substances that they contain may be contained in the list?
1. Products for use as mouthwashes
2. Products for use as eye ointments
3. Products for use for irrigation of wounds

Question 6
Which of the following items would not be allowed to be
classified as a GSL medicine?
1. Ovex – a tablet for the treatment of threadworms
2. Opticrom – an eyedrop used to alleviate the symptoms of
    hayfever
3. Anusol suppositories – used to treat haemorrhoids

Question 7
Which of the following statements concerning SOPs is true?
1. Originally designed to ensure clinical governance of the
    dispensing procedure.
2. An SOP for the dispensing procedure would be the same for
    every community pharmacy in a particular primary care
    trust.
3. An SOP for the dispensing procedure would NOT be
    required in hospital pharmacy because they are covered by
    Crown immunity.

Question 8
Which ONE of the following is NOT one of the seven essential
services as identified by the new pharmacy contract?
A   Dispensing
B   Counter prescribing
C   Disposal of unwanted medicines
D   Signposting
E   Promotion of healthy lifestyle

Question 9

Paracetamol may be a GSL, P or POM medicinal product. Which **ONE** of the following could **NOT** be considered a GSL medicine under any circumstances?

A   16 paracetamol effervescent tablets 500 mg
B   30 paracetamol effervescent tablets 120 mg
C   100 paracetamol effervescent tablets 500 mg
D   32 paracetamol tablets 500 mg
E   100 paracetamol tablets 500 mg

Question 10

Regarding the sale of naproxen as a pharmacy (P) medicine, which **ONE** of the following statements is true?

A   It can be sold for use in patients aged between 12 and 50.
B   Packs must NOT contain more than 5 days' supply.
C   The maximum daily dose is 1000 mg.
D   The maximum single dose is 500 mg.
E   It is indicated for the treatment of musculoskeletal pain and inflammation.

Question 11

Regarding the sale of hydrocortisone for external use as a GSL medicine, which **ONE** of the following statements is true?

A   A tube of ointment with a maximum strength of 1% would be suitable for a GSL sale.
B   The size of the tube of ointment or cream sold as a GSL medicine is 15 g.
C   It is indicated to treat reactions to insect bites and stings.
D   Its use is restricted to adults and children aged over 12 years.
E   Maximum length of treatment is 7 days.

Question 12

Regarding the classification of medicines which **ONE** of the following statements is true?

A   There is a definitive list of P medicines.
B   It is not a legal requirement for 64 paracetamol tablets to be sold by, or under the supervision of, a pharmacist.
C   Hypromellose eyedrops BPC (artificial tears) may be sold while the pharmacist is out at lunch.
D   A P medicine may be sold from any supermarket where a pharmacist is present to supervise the sale.
E   All homeopathic preparations that have a certificate of registration can be sold as if they had been given GSL status.

Summary

This chapter has introduced the text and explained the contents of the subsequent chapters. In addition, basic medicines classification has been described, where medicines are classified into three categories: GSL medicines, P medicines and POMs. Finally, the purpose and construction of SOPs have been covered.

It is important that student pharmacists and pharmacy technicians understand the points covered in this chapter and attempt the questions at the end of the chapter before moving on to any subsequent parts of the book.

chapter 2
NHS supply in the community 1: prescription forms and prescribing

Overview

Upon completion of this chapter, you should be able to:

- understand the mechanisms of supply of prescription items via the NHS in the community
- list the different pieces of information that need to be present on NHS prescription forms
- understand the purpose of the different UK *Drug Tariffs*
- define the types of items that may and may not be prescribed on an NHS prescription form
- understand the general restrictions that apply to the supply of items via an NHS prescription form.

Introduction and overview

This chapter provides an overview of the supply of prescription items via the National Health Service (NHS) in the community. Chapter 3 provides an overview of the different types of NHS prescribers and the dispensing process in the community.

The NHS is the publicly funded healthcare system for England. The devolved administrations of the UK countries are responsible for healthcare in their respective countries. The equivalent organisations in the other countries are called Health and Social Care in Northern Ireland, NHS Scotland and NHS Wales. For the purposes of this book, the term 'NHS' refers to all four healthcare organisations.

The following topics are covered in this chapter:
- NHS prescription supply
- supplies of prescription items via the NHS within the community
- the different UK *Drug Tariffs*
- items that may be prescribed on an NHS prescription form
- restrictions to supply on an NHS prescription form.

In addition to the supply of prescription items in the community (termed 'primary care'), items may also be supplied to patients within a hospital setting (termed 'secondary care'). The supply of items via the NHS within the hospital setting is covered in Chapter 4. (Items may also be supplied on prescription forms that are not part of the NHS, termed 'private prescriptions'. The supply of prescription items via private prescription forms is covered in Chapter 5.)

NHS prescription supply

Probably the most common form of prescription supply within community pharmacy is via an NHS prescription form. There are many different NHS prescription forms in use within the UK, but most follow a similar layout to that shown in Figures 2.1 (front) and 2.2 (back).

The differences between the prescription forms depend on whether the prescription is computer generated (which is more common nowadays) or handwritten, and the type of prescriber. In addition, there are differences between the prescription forms used for standard prescribing and those used

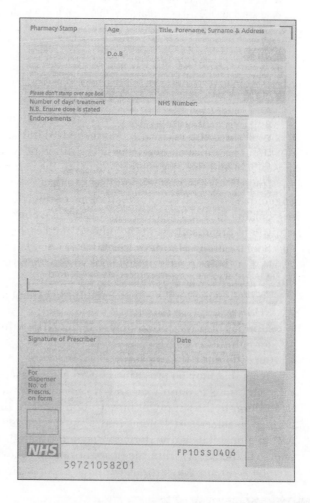

Figure 2.1 The front of a standard NHS prescription form (an FP10SS from England).

for instalment prescribing for addicts, which takes place on special larger prescription forms (the extra space is used to record the details of each instalment supplied). Further details on the prescribing for addicts can be found in Chapter 6.

In addition to the above, different prescription forms are used in the different countries that make up the UK. Although there are many variants, the different forms can be grouped as follows:

- FP10 – England
- HS21 – Northern Ireland (and HS21S for stock ordering)
- GP10 or HBP – Scotland (and GP10A for stock ordering)
- WP10 – Wales.

Stock ordering forms in Northern Ireland and Scotland are used by general practitioners to order stock drugs for use in their surgery (e.g. vaccines). There is no equivalent form for ordering stock in England and Wales.

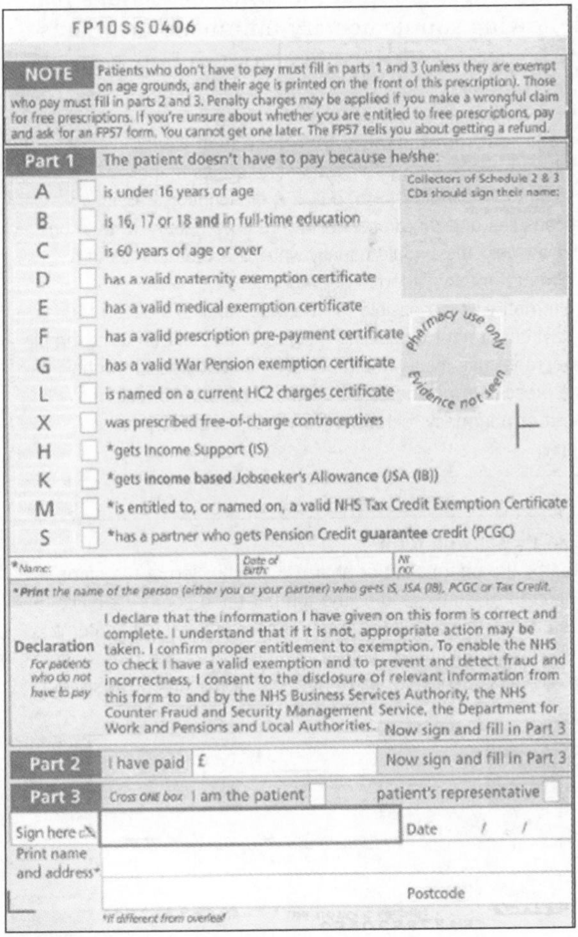
FP10SS0406

NOTE Patients who don't have to pay must fill in parts 1 and 3 (unless they are exempt on age grounds, and their age is printed on the front of this prescription). Those who pay must fill in parts 2 and 3. Penalty charges may be applied if you make a wrongful claim for free prescriptions. If you're unsure about whether you are entitled to free prescriptions, pay and ask for an FP57 form. You cannot get one later. The FP57 tells you about getting a refund.

Part 1 The patient doesn't have to pay because he/she:

Collectors of Schedule 2 & 3 CDs should sign their name:

A ☐ is under 16 years of age
B ☐ is 16, 17 or 18 and in full-time education
C ☐ is 60 years of age or over
D ☐ has a valid maternity exemption certificate
E ☐ has a valid medical exemption certificate
F ☐ has a valid prescription pre-payment certificate
G ☐ has a valid War Pension exemption certificate
L ☐ is named on a current HC2 charges certificate
X ☐ was prescribed free-of-charge contraceptives
H ☐ *gets Income Support (IS)
K ☐ *gets income based Jobseeker's Allowance (JSA (IB))
M ☐ *is entitled to, or named on, a valid NHS Tax Credit Exemption Certificate
S ☐ *has a partner who gets Pension Credit guarantee credit (PCGC)

Pharmacy use only — Evidence not seen

*Name: Date of Birth: NI No:

*Print the name of the person (either you or your partner) who gets IS, JSA (IB), PCGC or Tax Credit.

Declaration *For patients who do not have to pay* I declare that the information I have given on this form is correct and complete. I understand that if it is not, appropriate action may be taken. I confirm proper entitlement to exemption. To enable the NHS to check I have a valid exemption and to prevent and detect fraud and incorrectness, I consent to the disclosure of relevant information from this form to and by the NHS Business Services Authority, the NHS Counter Fraud and Security Management Service, the Department for Work and Pensions and Local Authorities. Now sign and fill in Part 3

Part 2 I have paid £ Now sign and fill in Part 3

Part 3 *Cross ONE box* I am the patient ☐ patient's representative ☐

Sign here Date / /

Print name and address*

Postcode

*If different from overleaf

Figure 2.2 The reverse of a standard NHS prescription form (an FP10SS) from England).

There are also different forms for the Isle of Man (HS10), Jersey (H9) and Guernsey (PS6). There are many forms currently in use, and changes to the forms occur from time to time. A detailed summary of the main prescription forms used in the UK and their respective uses can be found in *Applied Pharmaceutical Practice* (Langley and Belcher, 2008).

General prescription layout

As can be seen from the previous sections, there are a large number of different prescription forms in use within the UK. However, the prescription forms all follow a basic similar layout (Figure 2.3).

The front of the prescription form records the patient's details and details of the medication being prescribed. Finally, the prescriber's details are included at the bottom. Prescription forms from independent and supplementary prescribers also indicate the type of prescriber on the prescription form.

In addition to the explanation of the different sections in Figure 2.3, the following supplementary information explains the function of two specific sections of a prescription form.

Number of days' treatment (note: ensure that dose is stated)

It is usual for prescribers to write the quantity of each item to be prescribed alongside the item on the prescription form, e.g. if a prescription was for amoxicillin 250 mg capsules and the prescriber wanted the patient to take one three times a day for a week, they would usually write '21' (sometimes in a circle) or 'mitte 21' ('mitte' means 'send' – see Appendix 2).

However, as an alternative, it is possible for the prescriber to indicate the desired number of days' treatment by placing a figure in this box (in the example in the preceding paragraph, this figure would be '7'). As indicated in the box, it is important that the prescriber include a dose with each prescribed item to enable the pharmacist or pharmacy technician to calculate the number of dosage units to supply.

For dispenser No. of Prescns on form

This box is completed by the pharmacist or pharmacy technician at the same time as the prescription form is stamped at the top left-hand corner (see Figure 2.3). The figure entered into this box is the total number of prescription items on the form. This figure includes any items that attract more than one prescription charge (e.g. surgical stockings, some types of hormone replacement treatment [HRT]).

Figure 2.3 The layout of a standard NHS prescription form with an indication of where different pieces of information are located.

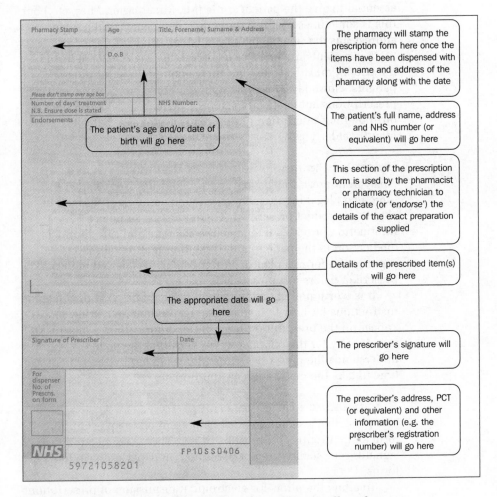

It is worth noting at this point that the public usually refer to the form in Figure 2.1 as 'a prescription'. Technically speaking a prescription is each item that is written on the form. Therefore, each *prescription form* can contain more than one *prescription*.

On the reverse of the prescription form, the patient or patient's representative completes the form to indicate whether the patient is exempt from prescription charges (and, if so, what exemption) or an indication of the number of prescription charges paid (see Figure 2.2).

NHS prescription form requirements

All NHS prescription forms require certain pieces of information to be present. These are as follows (see also Figure 2.3).

The patient's details

The name and address of the patient must be given. It is not essential to give the patient's title (Mr, Mrs, Master, Miss, etc.) but this is sometimes useful if more than one person at the same address has the same name (e.g. a father and son).

For patients under 12 years of age, the age *or* date of birth of the patient must be stated but this is not required for older patients. Nowadays, many computer systems used for generating prescriptions automatically print the patient's age and/or date of birth on the prescription form. This is useful as it helps to identify elderly patients.

Details of the medication to be supplied

Apart from prescribing some controlled drugs (see Chapter 6) there is no legal requirement to provide particular information about the product prescribed. There must be sufficient information provided to enable the accurate and safe supply of medication to the patient and, if the information on the prescription form is insufficient, this must be queried with the prescriber before a supply can be made.

It is worth noting that, although it would be good practice, the instructions for how to take or use the product do not have to appear on the prescription form. If this information is missing, it is necessary for the pharmacist to check that the patient understands the prescriber's intentions and advise the patient how to take the medication as appropriate.

The signature of the prescriber

The prescriber's signature must be present on the prescription form and currently this must be in ink. Therefore, electronic signatures or stamps are not permitted on paper prescription forms.

To allow the pilots for electronic transmission of prescriptions (ETP) to go ahead in England, the Prescription Only Medicines Order was amended to allow authorised prescribers who were participating in the pilot schemes to sign prescription forms digitally in place of ink signatures.

The address of the prescriber

The prescriber's address, which for most prescribers is usually the practice address, is pre-printed on the prescription form (along with details of the primary care organisation [PCT or equivalent] to which the practice belongs). For a nurse employed by a primary care organisation (as opposed to one employed by a surgery), the trust's address is printed on the form and the nurse has to add a code that identifies the patient's GP practice.

An indication of the prescriber type

Particulars to indicate whether the prescriber is a doctor, dentist, nurse, pharmacist or other prescriber need to be included on the prescription form. This does not have to be (and indeed on an NHS prescription form usually isn't) the prescriber's qualifications. NHS prescription forms are usually printed with a number to identify the prescriber.

An appropriate date

A date must appear on the prescription form next to the prescriber's signature. For most prescriptions this is the date that the prescriber signed the prescription form but the prescriber is also allowed to put a date before which the prescription should not be dispensed.

Post-dated prescription forms are used to prevent patients stockpiling large quantities of medication at home. For example, instead of providing one prescription form for 3 months' supply, the prescriber could give a patient three appropriately dated prescription forms, each for 1 month's supply. This results in the patient having less medication at home (as each supply of medication from the pharmacy would be only for a month) while still saving the patient from visiting the surgery each month.

The British National Formulary

The *BNF* contains advice for prescribers on how to write both handwritten and computer-generated prescriptions clearly.

Any prescriptions that do not contain the necessary information, or are unclear or ambiguous, need to be referred back to the prescriber for clarification.

KeyPoints

NHS prescription forms need the following pieces of information to be present:

- the patient's details
- details of the medication to be supplied
- the signature of the prescriber
- the address of the prescriber
- an indication of the prescriber type
- an appropriate date.

The *Drug Tariffs*

One of the most important non-clinical reference sources for the supply of items on an NHS prescription form is the *Drug Tariff*. Produced monthly, the *Drug Tariff* is the guide to what can and cannot be prescribed on an NHS prescription form. In addition, it also provides information on the amount that pharmacies will be reimbursed and remunerated for dispensing items on NHS prescription forms and performing other NHS services.

It should be noted that three separate *Drug Tariffs* exist (one for England and Wales, one for Northern Ireland and one for Scotland) and, although similar in nature, the contents and the layout of the different sections do differ among the three.

The *Drug Tariff* is probably not the easiest book to use and navigate your way around; however, it is vital that pharmacists and pharmacy technicians involved in the dispensing process be familiar with its layout. There are different classes of individuals who supply items against NHS prescriptions (pharmacists, dispensing doctors and appliance contractors) and so the *Drug Tariff* contains information for all three types of supplier (i.e. it is not solely a reference source for pharmacists and pharmacy technicians).

It is suggested that student pharmacists and pharmacy technicians either obtain a paper copy of the *Drug Tariff* or (for England and Wales only) access the contents online via the Prescription Pricing Division (PPD) website (part of the NHS Business Services Authority – see Bibliography). Unlike the online versions of many pharmaceutical texts, the online version of the *Drug Tariff for England and Wales* mirrors the paper version in both content and layout and so it can be used to learn how to navigate around the various parts of the paper version. There are also online versions of the *Scottish Drug Tariff* and the *Northern Ireland Drug Tariff.*

Notes on charges

In principle, in England and Scotland (although plans are in place to abolish prescription charges in Scotland), one prescription charge is payable for each prescription item. This charge is fixed and irrespective of the cost of the item or the number of dosage units. Patients who are not exempt from paying prescription charges are charged one prescription charge per item (this is not the case in Wales where all prescription items are free if prescribed via an NHS prescription form).

Although initially this would appear straightforward, there are a number of more complex charging scenarios that may occur. It is important that pharmacists and pharmacy technicians are aware of these different scenarios to ensure that they charge patients the correct amount.

This is important because the pharmacy is acting on behalf of the NHS in collecting the prescription charges. As the pharmacy keeps these charges, the Prescription Pricing Division deducts the amount collected from the monies that are paid to the pharmacy at the end of the month. This deduction is based on what the pharmacy *should* have collected, irrespective of what they *did* collect. Therefore, if a pharmacy does not take the correct number of prescription charges, they are financially disadvantaged. This is especially important

KeyPoint

In England, one prescription charge is payable for each prescription item. This charge is fixed and irrespective of the cost of the item or the number of dosage units.

for preparations containing more than one medicinal product (e.g. tablets for HRT where there may be 21 tablets containing one drug and 7 containing a different drug in the same packet). These preparations attract more than one prescription charge because, although there is only one 'box', there is more than one preparation within.

A summary of the charging rules is as follows.

Single prescription charge payable

- The same drug or preparation is supplied in more than one container.
- Different strengths of the same drug in the same formulation are ordered as separate prescriptions on the same prescription form.
- More than one appliance of the same type (other than hosiery*) is supplied.
- A set of parts making up a complete appliance is supplied.
- Drugs are supplied in powder form with the solvent separate for subsequent admixing.
- A drug is supplied with a dropper, throat brush or vaginal applicator.
- Several flavours of the same preparation are supplied.

Multiple prescription charges payable

- Different drugs, types of dressing or appliances are supplied.
- Different formulations or presentations of the same drug or preparation are prescribed and supplied.
- Additional parts are supplied together with a complete set of apparatus or additional dressing(s) together with a dressing pack.
- More than one piece of elastic hosiery* is supplied, e.g. two stockings are a pair and will attract two charges.

*Anklet, legging, knee-cap, below-knee, above-knee or thigh stocking.

> **KeyPoint**
>
> There are a number of situations where a single prescription item attracts more than one prescription charge. Student pharmacists and pharmacy technicians should ensure that they become familiar with the different charging models.

Items that may be prescribed on an NHS prescription form

For ease of understanding, it is best to separate prescribing of items on an NHS prescription form into three categories:

1. medicinal products (i.e. drugs)
2. appliances (e.g. stoma equipment)
3. chemical reagents (e.g. test strips for diabetes).

KeyPoint

All medicinal products may be prescribed on an NHS prescription form, provided that the prescriber is authorised to prescribe that item and the item is not subject to any specific restrictions.

KeyPoint

Only those appliances listed within the respective *Drug Tariff* may be prescribed on an NHS prescription form.

Medicinal products

All medicinal products may be prescribed on an NHS prescription form (provided that the prescriber is authorised to prescribe that item) so long as the item is not subject to any specific restrictions.

Appliances

Only those appliances listed within the respective *Drug Tariff* may be prescribed on an NHS prescription form. If an appliance is not listed, it may not be prescribed on an NHS prescription form and, if pharmacists dispense an appliance not listed within the *Drug Tariff*, they would not be reimbursed the cost of the item.

All approved appliances for England and Wales can be found in Part IX of the *Drug Tariff*:

- Part IXA contains an alphabetical list of appliances (e.g. atomisers, peak flow meters) and dressings that are allowed to be prescribed on an NHS prescription form. All items included in Part IXA are listed in the index at the back of the *Drug Tariff*.
- Part IXB contains a list of incontinence appliances that can be prescribed on an NHS prescription form. At the front of Part IXB there is an index of component headings, and each section thereafter is listed alphabetically by manufacturer's name.
- Part IXC contains a list of stoma appliances that can be prescribed on an NHS prescription form. The format of this section follows the same pattern as for Part IXB.

The *Northern Ireland Drug Tariff* lists approved appliances in Part III and similar lists can be found in the *Scottish Drug Tariff*. Each Part of the *Scottish Drug Tariff* starts with an alphabetical list of product types and, within each type, individual products are listed in alphabetical order:

- Part 2 – dressings
- Part 3 – appliances
- Part 4 – elastic hosiery
- Part 5 – incontinence appliances
- Part 6 – stoma appliances.

Chemical reagents

As with the prescribing of appliances, the only chemical reagents that may be prescribed on an NHS prescription form are those listed within the respective *Drug Tariff*. If a reagent is not listed, it may not be prescribed on an NHS prescription and, if pharmacists dispense a reagent not listed within the *Drug Tariff*, they would not be reimbursed the cost of the item.

KeyPoint

Only those chemical reagents listed within the respective *Drug Tariff* may be prescribed on an NHS prescription form.

In England and Wales, all approved reagents can be found in Part IXR of the *Drug Tariff*. A sentence at the start of this section explains the order in which the products are listed. They are also listed by brand name in the index at the back of the *Drug Tariff*. For Northern Ireland all approved reagents can be found in Part II of the *Northern Ireland Drug Tariff* and, for Scotland, in Part 9 of the *Scottish Drug Tariff*.

Restrictions to supply on an NHS prescription form

In addition to any clinical and patient-specific issues that need to be taken into consideration when supplying an item against a prescription, there are a number of additional restrictions that are placed upon certain items being prescribed (and therefore dispensed) on an NHS prescription form. It should be remembered that these restrictions are based on the nature of the item and specific to NHS prescription forms (i.e. the item may be prescribed on a private prescription form – see Chapter 5).

Appropriate prescribers may prescribe any medicinal product on an NHS prescription form, within their approved areas, unless it is prohibited by the *Drug Tariff*. These restrictions can be divided into three groups:
1. borderline substances (ACBS restrictions)
2. drugs and other substances not to be prescribed under the NHS Pharmaceutical Services
3. drugs to be prescribed in certain circumstances under the NHS Pharmaceutical Services (SLS restrictions).

Borderline substances
Details of borderline substances can be found in Part XV of the *Drug Tariff for England and Wales* and Part X of the *Northern Ireland Drug Tariff*. Information can also be found in Appendix 7 of the *British National Formulary*.

Borderline substances are described by the *Drug Tariff for England and Wales* as follows:

> In certain conditions some foods and toilet preparations have characteristics of drugs and the Advisory Committee on Borderline Substances advises as to the circumstances in which such substances may be regarded as drugs.

Therefore, these items are not drugs as such; they are foods or toiletries that may in certain circumstances be prescribed on an NHS prescription form.

The relevant Part of the *Drug Tariffs* is divided into two lists: List A and List B. List A gives an alphabetical index of products that the Advisory Committee on Borderline Substances (ACBS) has recommended for the management of the conditions shown under each product. List B is a cross index listing clinical conditions and the products that the ACBS has approved for the management of those conditions. It is normal to consult List A first.

So, for an item in List A of Part XV of the *Drug Tariff for England and Wales* (or equivalent) to be prescribed on an NHS prescription form, the patient should be being treated for a listed condition. To indicate that this criterion has been met, the prescriber should endorse the prescription 'ACBS'. Pharmacists may dispense any item listed in Part XV of the *Drug Tariff for England and Wales* (or equivalent) even if it has not been endorsed 'ACBS' by the prescriber. However, items listed in Part XV of the *Drug Tariff* that are not endorsed 'ACBS' by the prescriber may result in the prescriber being asked by the PCT (or equivalent) to justify why the product has been supplied at NHS expense.

It is important that pharmacists are aware of the contents of the relevant Part of the *Drug Tariff*. Each *Drug Tariff* is updated on a monthly basis and so is the primary reference source for information on borderline substances. However, the *British National Formulary* also indicates whether an item would need to be endorsed 'ACBS' before being supplied by listing the various products in Appendix 7.

Pharmacists and pharmacy technicians should always remember that the *British National Formulary* is updated only once every 6 months and so is usually less up to date than the *Drug Tariff*. Therefore, wherever possible pharmacists and pharmacy technicians should use their respective *Drug Tariff* for information on borderline substances.

KeyPoints

Borderline substances are foods or toiletries that may in certain circumstances be prescribed on an NHS prescription form.

For items on the borderline substances list, the prescriber should endorse the prescription 'ACBS' to indicate that the patient is being treated for a listed condition.

Drugs and other substances not to be prescribed under the NHS Pharmaceutical Services

Part XVIIIA of the *Drug Tariff for England and Wales* and Part XIA of the *Northern Ireland Drug Tariff* list those drugs and other substances not to be prescribed on an NHS prescription form. These sections were colloquially referred to as the 'Black List', although this is a term that is not used much nowadays. Similar information for Scotland is contained in Schedule 10 to the NHS (General Medical Services) Regulations 1992.

If a medicinal product appears on this list, it cannot be prescribed on an NHS prescription form (and therefore should not be dispensed). Many of the items on this list are proprietary items, e.g. Calpol Infant Suspension. However, so long as the generic name for the items does not also appear on the list, the item may be prescribed generically.

It is important that pharmacists are aware of the contents of the respective Parts of their *Drug Tariff*. The *Drug Tariff* is updated on a monthly basis and so is the primary reference source for information on items which are not to be prescribed on an NHS prescription form. However, the *British National Formulary* also indicates whether an item is not to be prescribed on the NHS by annotating the monograph in the text with a crossed-out 'NHS' (Figure 2.4). However, pharmacists and pharmacy technicians should always remember that the *British National Formulary* is updated only once every 6 months and so is usually less up to date than the respective *Drug Tariff*.

KeyPoint

Each *Drug Tariff* lists those items that must not be prescribed on an NHS prescription form. These lists were colloquially referred to as the 'Black List'.

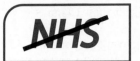

Figure 2.4 This entry next to an item's monograph in the *British National Formulary* indicates that it is not to be prescribed on an NHS prescription form.

Drugs to be prescribed in certain circumstances under the NHS Pharmaceutical Services (SLS restrictions)

Part XVIIIA of the *Drug Tariff for England and Wales*, Part XIB of the *Northern Ireland Drug Tariff* and Part 12 of the *Scottish Drug Tariff* list those drugs that may be prescribed only on an NHS prescription form for certain conditions or certain patients, along with a list of those conditions and/or patients. This section is similar to borderline substances (see above) except there we are dealing with items that may or may not have been prescribed for medical reasons (i.e. foods and toiletries). In this case, the items are all drugs, but they may be prescribed only in certain conditions or for certain patients.

To indicate that the criteria within this Part of the *Drug Tariff* have been met, the prescriber must endorse the prescription 'SLS' (Selective List Scheme) (or 'S.11' in Northern Ireland). Pharmacists should not dispense any item listed in these respective Parts of the *Drug Tariff* unless it has been endorsed 'SLS' (or 'S.11') by the prescriber. It is not the role of the pharmacist to verify that the patient is indeed being treated for a listed condition; this is the responsibility of the prescriber.

It is important that pharmacists are aware of the contents of the respective Parts of their *Drug Tariff*. The *Drug Tariff* is updated on a monthly basis and so is the primary reference source for information on 'SLS' restrictions. However, the *British National Formulary* also indicates whether an item would need to be endorsed 'SLS' before being supplied by annotating the monograph in the text 'SLS' and adding footnotes. However, pharmacists and pharmacy technicians should always remember that the *British National Formulary* is updated only once every 6 months and so is usually less up to date than the respective *Drug Tariff*.

KeyPoints

In addition to borderline substances, each *Drug Tariff* lists those drugs that must be prescribed on an NHS prescription form only in certain circumstances.

The drugs and the circumstances in which they may be prescribed can be found in the respective *Drug Tariff*.

Worked examples

Example 2.1

Dr Villa is on the telephone. He has to write an NHS prescription for a patient of his with a rather nasty wound. He would like some Sorbsan flat dressings but he is not sure which size they come in. He definitely needs something bigger than 10 cm × 20 cm. Can you advise him?

This is the largest Sorbsan flat dressing available on the NHS. It is an alginate dressing for wounds with medium-to-heavy exudation (see the *Drug Tariff for England and Wales*, Part IXA).

Alternative larger alginate dressings allowed on the NHS include Algisite M 15 cm × 20 cm, Curasorb 15 cm × 25 cm and 30 cm × 61 cm, and Kaltostat 15 cm × 25 cm.

Example 2.2

Dr Villa is on the telephone. He has to write an NHS prescription for a patient of his who has requested some Sudafed Linctus (she is a senior citizen and therefore does not pay an NHS charge). He has never prescribed this before. Is there anything that he should know and how should he proceed?

Advise Dr Villa that Sudafed Linctus is blacklisted. It consists of a mixture of pseudoephedrine 30 mg and dextromethorphan 10 mg/5 mL.

Suggest that he could achieve the same treatment using pseudoephedrine elixir and pholcodine linctus, as both are allowed on an NHS prescription.

Self-assessment

For questions 1–4 below, **ONE** or **MORE** of the responses/statements is/are correct. Decide which of the responses/statements is/are correct and then choose:
A   If statements 1, 2 and 3 are all correct
B   If statements 1 and 2 are correct and statement 3 is incorrect
C   If statements 2 and 3 are correct and statement 1 is incorrect
D   If statement 1 is correct and statements 2 and 3 are incorrect
E   If statement 3 is correct and statements 1 and 2 are incorrect

Question 1
What is specified on the back of an FP10 prescription form?
1.   **Exemption categories for patients who do not pay the prescription charge**
2.   **The patient's home address**
3.   **The name and address of the prescriber**

Question 2
Which of the following NHS prescription forms can be used to prescribe in instalments?
1.   **FP10MDA-SS**
2.   **FP10MDA-S**
3.   **FP10SS**

Question 3
Consider the following statements about borderline substances. Which are correct?
1.   **Borderline substances are foods and cosmetics that have been approved for the treatment of specific medical conditions.**
2.   **A pharmacist will always be paid for an ACBS item whether or not the prescriber has indicated 'ACBS' on the prescription.**
3.   **If the prescription is NOT endorsed 'ACBS' by the prescriber, the pharmacist may add the endorsement.**

Question 4
A prescriber has to include the following on an FP10 prescription in order to meet legal requirements.
1.   **Prescriber's signature**
2.   **Patient's home address**
3.   **The instructions to the patient as to how to use or take the medicine**

Question 5

With regard to NHS prescriptions, which **ONE** of the following statements is true?

A   It is a legal requirement that the age of the patient be given on all prescription forms for a POM medicine.

B   A prescriber may indicate instalment prescribing on an FP10NC.

C   It is a legal requirement that all prescriptions for a prescription-only medicine contain an appropriate date.

D   A doctor may write a single prescription for a POM to treat more than one patient in the same family.

E   A doctor can prescribe any chemical reagent on an NHS prescription.

Question 6

Regarding NHS prescribers and prescriptions which **ONE** of the following statements is true?

A   A community practitioner nurse prescriber may prescribe any licensed POM for any medical condition within their area of competence.

B   A registered dentist can prescribe any licensed POM on an NHS prescription.

C   A practitioner may include instruction on an NHS prescription to allow for repeat dispensing of the same prescription.

D   When writing an NHS prescription a practitioner may use carbon paper to make a number of copies; each will be valid provided that the prescriber signs each copy of the prescription in indelible ink.

E   Pharmacist independent prescribers may prescribe any licensed POM within their area of competence.

For questions 7–14 below, select the **ONE** response from A–E below as the number of prescription charges that are payable for an NHS prescription presented by a patient who is **NOT** exempt from prescription charges.

A   0 charges

B   1 charge

C   2 charges

D   3 charges

E   4 charges

Question 7

How many charges would be applicable for a prescription form for the following items?

28 phenoxymethylpenicillin 250 mg tablets
28 warfarin 1 mg tablets
28 warfarin 3 mg tablets
28 warfarin 5 mg tablets

Question 8

How many prescription charges would be applicable if two
prescription forms were received, both for the same patient,
where the first prescription form was for:

28 penicillin V tablets
28 warfarin 1 mg tablets

and the second was for:

28 warfarin 3 mg tablets
28 warfarin 5 mg tablets

Question 9

How many charges would be applicable for a prescription form
for the following items?
63 Microgynon 30 tablets
1 salbutamol inhaler 100 micrograms MDI
1 beclometasone 200 micrograms MDI

Question 10

How many charges would be applicable for a prescription form
for the following items?
28 dosulepin 25 mg capsules
28 dosulepin 75 mg tablets

Question 11

How many charges would be applicable for a prescription form
for the following item?
1 × OP Premique Cycle Calendar Pack

Question 12

How many charges would be applicable for a prescription form
for the following items?
1 × OP Premique tablet

Question 13

How many charges would be applicable for a prescription form
for the following items?
100 co-dydramol tablets
84 diclofenac 50 mg tablets
1 pair of anklets class II

Question 14

How many charges would be applicable for a prescription form for the following items?

Fortisip Multi Fibre strawberry 3 × 200 mL
Fortisip Multi Fibre orange 3 × 200 mL
Fortisip Multi Fibre banana 3 × 200 mL
Fortijuce blackcurrant 3 × 200 mL

Summary

This chapter has recapped on the key basics behind the supply of medication via an NHS prescription form in the community. It is important that these concepts are understood before the student pharmacist or pharmacy technician tackles the actual mechanics of medicines supply via the NHS in the community. The application of these concepts to the supply of medicinal products via NHS prescription forms in the community is dealt with in Chapter 3.

chapter 3

NHS supply in the community 2: prescribers and the dispensing process

Overview

Upon completion of this chapter, you should be able to:
- list which types of prescriber may prescribe items via an NHS prescription form and what restrictions are placed on each type of prescriber
- summarise the general dispensing procedure for NHS prescriptions in the community
- complete a number of worked examples and self-assessment questions involving NHS prescriptions and the dispensing process.

Introduction and overview

The material in this chapter follows on from Chapter 2, by covering the supply of prescription items via the National Health Service (NHS) in the community. The following topics are covered:
- NHS prescribers
- the dispensing procedure for NHS prescriptions
- a collection of worked examples and self-assessment questions
- a chapter summary.

NHS prescribers

NHS prescriptions are written by the following groups of prescribers:
- doctors
- dentists
- nurse prescribers
- supplementary prescribers
- independent non-medical prescribers.

Each of these different prescribers has different restrictions as to what he or she may prescribe on an NHS prescription form.

KeyPoints

NHS prescriptions can be written by:
- doctors
- dentists
- nurses
- supplementary prescribers
- independent non-medical pre-scribers.

Different restrictions on what may be prescribed on an NHS prescription form apply to different prescribers.

Details on the different restrictions can be found in *Applied Pharmaceutical Practice* (Langley and Belcher, 2008) (section 3.2).

The dispensing procedure for NHS prescriptions

Upon receipt of an NHS prescription form, the following procedure should be followed:

1. Check the legality of the NHS prescription form.
2. Identify the prescriber.
3. Check that the prescriber is allowed to prescribe the item(s) on an NHS prescription form.
4. Perform a clinical check on the prescription.
5. Dispense and label the item(s).
6. Check that the item(s) dispensed is/are correct and labelled appropriately; ideally this check would be performed by a colleague (i.e. an independent check) but, when working alone, the pharmacist needs to check the item(s) him- or herself.
7. Pass the item(s) to the patient and counsel him or her in the use of the medication.
8. Process the prescription form.

KeyPoints

The dispensing procedure for NHS prescriptions:
1. Check the legality of the NHS prescription form
2. Identify the prescriber
3. Check that the prescriber is allowed to prescribe the item(s) on an NHS prescription form
4. Perform a clinical check on the prescription
5. Dispense and label the item(s)
6. Check that the item(s) dispensed is/are correct and labelled appropriately
7. Pass the item(s) to the patient and counsel him or her in the use of the medication
8. Process the prescription form.

Further details on the individual parts of the dispensing procedure can be found in *Applied Pharmaceutical Practice* (Langley and Belcher 2008) (section 3.3).

Worked examples

Although a number of different examples are used in this section, from a variety of different prescribers, all prescription forms can be addressed by using a standard systematic approach.

Framework for systematic dispensing/supply in the community (Figure 3.1)

Example 3.1

You receive the prescription in Figure 3.2 in your pharmacy.

1. Identity of order

NHS prescription (FP10D).

2. Prescriber

Dentist.

Figure 3.1 Framework for systematic dispensing/supply in the community. (Continued overleaf)

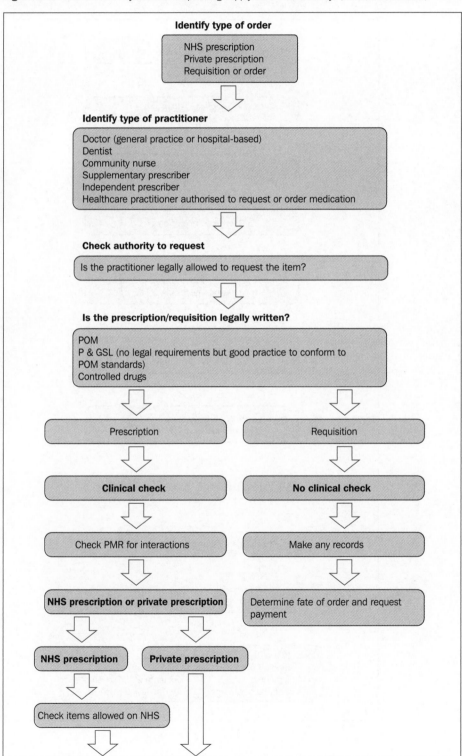

Figure 3.1 continued

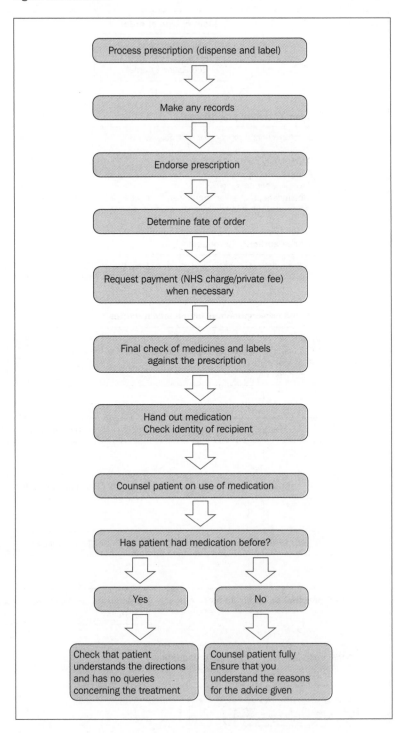

Figure 3.2

```
Pharmacy Stamp    | Age          | Title, Forename, Surname & Address
                  |              |
                  | D.o.B        | Mr Harry Baker
                  |              | 54 Somerset Place
                  | 01/08/63     | Anytown
                  |              | AT7 6SP
Please don't stamp over age box
Number of days' treatment        | NHS Number:  1234567890
N.B. Ensure dose is stated
Endorsements


        Co amoxiclav tablets
                     250/125


        1 tds


        Mitte 21                              FP10D0406




Signature of Dentist              | Date
W E Drillett                      | Today's

For         | Dentist's name and address
dispenser   |
No. of      | W. E. Drillett Anytown PCT
Prescns.    |
on form     | Anytown Dental Surgery       789123
            | ANYTOWN
            | AN1 2RB
            | 01674 536343
NHS                                 FP10D0406
```

3. Legally written?

Yes.

4. Clinical check (complete Table 3.1)

Table 3.1

Drug	Indications	Dose check	Reference
Co-amoxiclav	Severe dental infections with spreading cellulitis	Expressed as amoxicillin 250 mg every 8 h for 5 days	British National Formulary, 56th edn, section 5.1.1
Amoxicillin	Oral infections	250 mg every 8 h, doubled in severe infections	British National Formulary, 56th edn, section 5.1.1

5. Interactions

There is only one item on the prescription form. However, it would also be advisable for the pharmacist or pharmacy technician to check the patient's medication record (PMR) for any concurrent medication that could cause an interaction. In this case, the PMR indicated that there were no interactions with any previous or concurrent medication.

6. Suitability for patient
The item prescribed is safe and suitable for an adult patient and the dose ordered on the prescription is within the recommended dose limits.

7. Item(s) allowable on the NHS
No. The *Dental Practitioner's Formulary* indicates that dentists are not allowed to prescribe co-amoxiclav on an NHS prescription form.

Return prescription to the dentist for alteration to allowable item such as amoxicillin 250 mg capsules with a suggested dose of 250 mg every 8 hours for 5 days

8. Records to be made (including copies of the record[s])
Make a note of the intervention on a clinical intervention form (for an example of a clinical intervention form see *Applied Pharmaceutical Practice* (Langley and Belcher, 2008), Figure 1.5a.

9. Process prescription (including example of label[s])
- Prepare a label
- Check appendix 9 of the *British National Formulary* for supplementary labelling requirements:
  Amoxicillin: *British National Formulary* label number 9 (Take at regular intervals. Complete the prescribed course unless otherwise directed)
- Select amoxicillin capsules from shelf, remembering to check expiry date
- Perform final check of item, label and prescription
- Pack in a suitable bag ready to give to patient/patient's representative.

Labels (we have assumed that the name and address of the pharmacy and the words 'Keep out of the reach and sight of children' are pre-printed on the label) (Figure 3.3).

Figure 3.3

Amoxicillin Capsules 250 mg	15
Take ONE capsule every EIGHT hours.	
Take at regular intervals.	
Complete the prescribed course unless otherwise directed.	
Mr Harry Baker	Date of dispensing

10. Endorse prescription
Stamp with pharmacy stamp to indicate completion.

11. Destination of paperwork

Send to the PPD (Prescription Pricing Division) at the end of the month.

12. Identity check/counselling

- Check patient's name and address
- Explain change in medication without alarming the patient
- Reinforce the dose of the medication; explain need to take the medication at regular intervals and to complete the prescribed course
- Draw patient's attention to the patient information leaflet (PIL) and ask if he has any questions.

Example 3.2

You receive the prescription in Figure 3.4 in your pharmacy.

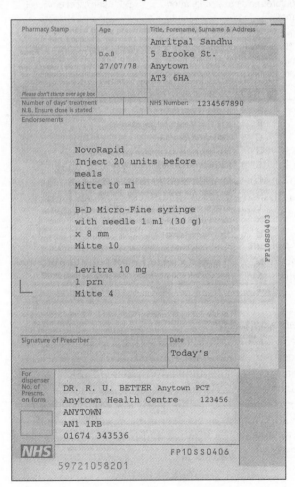

Figure 3.4

1. Identity of order
NHS prescription (FP10SS).

2. Prescriber
Doctor (general practitioner).

3. Legally written?
No signature; return prescription form to prescriber for addition of signature.

4. Clinical check (complete Table 3.2)

Table 3.2

Drug	Indications	Dose check	Reference
Insulin aspart	Diabetes mellitus	According to needs immediately before meals or shortly after meals	*British National Formulary* 56th edn, section 6.1.1
Vardenafil	Erectile dysfunction	Initially 10 mg approximately 25–30 min before sexual activity, subsequent doses adjusted according to response up to a max. 20 mg as a single dose	*British National Formulary* 56th edn, section 7.4.5

5. Interactions
The drugs on the prescription do not interact. However, it would also be advisable for the pharmacist or pharmacy technician to check the PMR for any concurrent medication that could cause an interaction. It should also be noted that plasma concentrations of vardenafil may be increased if taken with grapefruit juice.

6. Suitability for patient
The items prescribed are safe and suitable for an adult patient and the doses ordered on the prescription are within the recommended dose limits.

7. Item(s) allowable on the NHS
Yes (see *Drug Tariff for England and Wales*, Part XVIIB [Drugs to be prescribed in certain circumstances under NHS Pharmaceutical Services]). The medication ordered indicates that the patient has diabetes so Levitra may be prescribed under the selected list scheme. The prescription needs to be returned to the prescriber for the addition of an 'SLS' endorsement in the body of the prescription, next to the Levitra, so that it will be passed for payment by the PPD.

8. Records to be made (including copies of the record[s])
Make a note of the intervention on a clinical intervention form.

9. Process prescription (including example of label[s])
- Prepare a label for each product
- Check appendix 9 of the *British National Formulary* for supplementary labelling requirements (there are none)
- Select items from shelf, remembering to check expiry dates
- Perform final check of items, labels and prescription form
- Pack in a suitable bag ready to give to patient/patient's representative
- If patient/representative is not waiting ensure that the insulin is stored in the refrigerator until collected.

Labels (we have assumed that the name and address of the pharmacy and the words 'Keep out of the reach and sight of children' are pre-printed on the label) (Figures 3.5 and 3.6).

NovoRapid 100 U/mL	10 mL
Inject TWENTY units before meals.	
Store in fridge.	
Amritpal Sandhu	Date of dispensing

Figure 3.5

Levitra 10 mg Tablets	4
ONE to be taken when required.	
Amritpal Sandhu	Date of dispensing

Figure 3.6

The syringes do not legally have to be labelled but most pharmacies would label for stock control purposes (Figure 3.7).

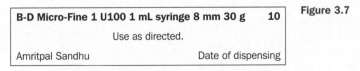

B-D Micro-Fine 1 U100 1 mL syringe 8 mm 30 g	10
Use as directed.	
Amritpal Sandhu	Date of dispensing

Figure 3.7

10. Endorse prescription
Stamp with pharmacy stamp to indicate completion.

11. Destination of paperwork
Send to the PPD at the end of the month.

12. Identity check/counselling
- Check patient's name and address
- Check that patient has had insulin before and is confident with its use
- Confirm that the insulin dispensed is the expected item

- Advise that the insulin should be refrigerated – it can be stored for up to 1 month at ambient temperatures
- Advise on how to take Levitra and explain that effects may persist for longer than 24 hours
- It is advisable to avoid grapefruit juice because it may interact with the Levitra
- It is also advisable to avoid fatty foods as these delay the onset of action of vardenafil
- Draw patient's attention to the PIL and ask if he has any questions.

Self-assessment

The following section of questions contains examples of NHS prescriptions that may be encountered in a community pharmacy. For each question, complete the following sections to guide you through the dispensing process:

1. identity of order
2. prescriber
3. legally written?
4. clinical check (complete Table 3.3).
5. interactions
6. suitability for patient
7. item(s) allowable on the NHS
8. records to be made (including copies of the record[s])
9. process prescription (including example of label[s]) – you may assume that any recommendations you may have made above have been acted upon by the prescriber
10. endorse prescription
11. destination of paperwork
12. identity check/counselling.

Table 3.3

Drug	Indications	Dose check	Reference

Question 1

You receive the prescription shown in Figure 3.8 in your pharmacy.

Using the sections indicated above, summarise all stages of the dispensing process for this prescription form.

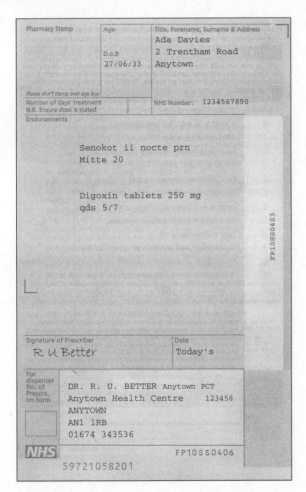

Figure 3.8

Question 2

You receive the prescription shown in Figure 3.9 in your pharmacy.

Using the sections indicated above, summarise all stages of the dispensing process for this prescription form.

Figure 3.9

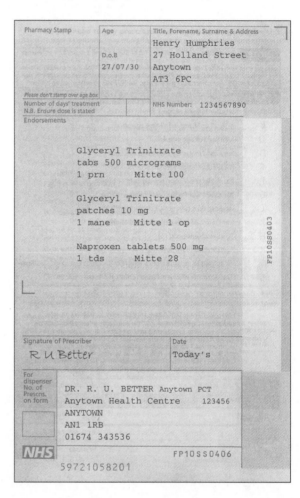

Question 3

You receive the prescription shown in Figure 3.10 in your pharmacy.

Using the sections indicated above, summarise all stages of the dispensing process for this prescription form.

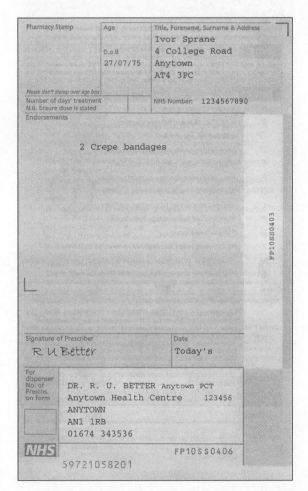

Figure 3.10

Question 4

You receive the prescription shown in Figure 3.11 in your pharmacy.

Using the sections indicated above, summarise all stages of the dispensing process for this prescription form.

Figure 3.11

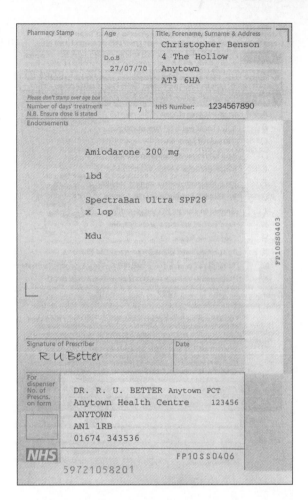

Summary

This chapter has taken the concepts covered in Chapter 2 and used them to discuss the points with which it is necessary to become familiar in order to supply medication via an NHS prescription form in the community. This includes details on the different prescribers who prescribe on NHS prescription forms and a discussion of the general dispensing procedure for NHS prescriptions in the community.

A collection of worked examples and self-assessment questions has been provided and it is suggested that the student pharmacist or pharmacy technician works though these exercises and ensures that they are familiar with the key learning points.

chapter 4
NHS supply within hospitals

Overview

Upon completion of this chapter, you should be able to:

■ understand the supply of medication to hospital inpatients including:
- inpatient drug charts
- discharge medications (TTOs/TTAs)
- patients' own drugs (PODs) schemes
- dispensing for discharge schemes
- self-medication schemes
■ understand the supply of medication to hospital outpatients
■ complete a number of worked examples and self-assessment exercises involving NHS hospital prescriptions and the dispensing process.

Introduction and overview

This chapter covers the supply of medicines via the National Health Service (NHS) within hospitals. Throughout this chapter, the term 'hospital' is used, but the types of supply described may also apply to other residential style care establishments, e.g. some care homes and hospices. It should be noted that the procedures discussed in this chapter for NHS hospitals are equally applicable to the supply of medication within a private sector establishment, the only difference being that the medication and care are entirely funded by the patient (or their healthcare insurance company).

The dispensing process within hospitals is similar in a number of ways to the supply of items on NHS prescriptions within community pharmacy (see Chapters 2 and 3). The main difference is that the supply is not usually on an NHS prescription form (except in some cases where the prescription originates from a prescriber within a hospital, but it is intended for it to be dispensed within the community).

Supply of medication within a hospital setting

The supply of medication by the pharmacy department within a hospital can be divided into three main categories:

1. inpatient supply
2. discharge medication
3. outpatient supply.

KeyPoints

The supply of medication by the pharmacy department within a hospital can be divided into three main categories:
1. inpatient supply
2. discharge medication
3. outpatient supply.

KeyPoints

Inpatient medication is an item ordered for a specific patient for use during his or her stay on the ward.

Inpatient orders are for medication not usually kept as 'stock' on the patient's ward.

Inpatient supply

Many patients admitted to hospital need some form of medication to be administered at some point during their stay, and details of this medication are made on the patient's inpatient drug chart. The type of medication supplied may depend on the reason for admission but patients may be on other medication that is not related to the reason for admission.

An inpatient order form usually specifies the name of the patient, the patient's ward, and the name and strength of the drug required. Note that the dosage of the drug is not usually specified on the order because this is detailed on the patient's drug chart. The dosage would be specified on the order (and therefore the label) only if the medication were being supplied as part of a *dispensing for discharge scheme*.

Discharge medication

Discharge medication is also termed TTO (*to take out*) or TTA (*to take away*) medication. This is the medication given to a patient on discharge. Enough medication is supplied (usually 14 days' supply) to allow for the discharge letter to be sent to the patient's general practitioner who then takes over the regular prescribing of the patient's medication. TTOs are written either on a specific section of the patient's drug chart or on hospital-specific forms. TTOs require the same information as any other prescription (including directions for administration for the patient to follow), the difference being that they may be dispensed only within the hospital.

KeyPoint

Discharge medication is also termed TTO (*to take out*) or TTA (*to take away*) medication, and is a hospital-based prescription for a specific patient used to provide the patient with a supply (usually 14 days) of medication upon discharge.

Patients' own drugs

More recently, changes in hospital procedures have allowed the use of drugs brought into hospital by patients. This not only prevents unnecessary wastage, but also reduces the hospital's drugs bill.

With a *patients' own drugs (POD) scheme*, patients still bring in their medication from home and this is then assessed by the ward pharmacist during the admission process. If there is sufficient medication left, in a suitable condition and labelled appropriately, this is added to the drugs trolley and used for that patient during drug rounds. In

KeyPoint

Patients' own drugs (POD) *schemes* allow the use of medication brought into the hospital by patients. The medication is checked by the ward pharmacists for suitability and the patient's drug chart annotated appropriately.

addition, on discharge, if there is still sufficient medication remaining and there has been no change to the dosage, etc., the medication is returned to the patient, rather than giving newly dispensed medication from the hospital pharmacy. Apart from the obvious cost savings, if all the medication that the patient is to be discharged on is his or her own, this also speeds up the discharge process.

Dispensing for discharge

In addition to POD schemes, another system recently introduced into hospital medication supply practice is the introduction of *dispensing for discharge schemes*. This is a combination of an inpatient order and a TTO. With this scheme, any medication required as an inpatient order is labelled as for a TTO. When the patient is then discharged, the medication and labelling are re-checked by the ward pharmacist and, if suitable, used as TTO medication.

> ## KeyPoints
>
> Dispensing for discharge schemes allow inpatient medication to be labelled for use upon discharge. Usually, in excess of 14 days' supply is provided to allow for use both during the patient's stay and on discharge.
>
> Before discharge, the ward pharmacists verify that the medication is still suitable for use (e.g. checking that the dose hasn't altered since original dispensing).

For this system to work effectively, more than 14 days' supply is usually provided in the first place to allow for both the inpatient and the TTO supply. This reduces the instances of items being dispensed twice for a patient (i.e. once as an inpatient order and once as a TTO) and therefore reduces both dispensing time and cost.

Self-medication schemes

Although different to POD schemes and dispensing for discharge schemes, the use of *self-medication schemes* is also worthy of mention. Here, instead of the medication being placed on the ward drugs trolley for administration by the nursing staff, the patient is given the medicine for self-administration (e.g. the medication may be kept in a locked cupboard by the patient's bed and a key given to the patient).

Patients operating within this scheme are first assessed for suitability (usually by the ward pharmacist). Although this scheme would not be suitable for all patients, there are a significant number of patients who are perfectly capable of self-administering medication. This not only enables a patient to be in control of his or her own medication, but also helps to reduce staff workload.

Outpatient supply

Patients also visit a hospital for outpatient appointments: the patient comes to the hospital to see a specialist, usually in a specific clinic. Depending on the individual circumstances, an outpatient may require a supply of prescribed drugs. This prescribing is usually the role of the patient's GP; however, as with prescribing TTO medication, it may take time for the details of the prescribed medication to reach the patient's GP by letter.

In these circumstances, it may be necessary for the hospital doctor to provide a supply of the medication. This is usually achieved via an internal outpatient supply form, which can be dispensed only within the hospital pharmacy. Outpatient supply forms are specific to each hospital and contain the same type of information as an NHS prescription form.

Although it is usual for any prescriptions issued by hospital prescribers to outpatients to be dispensed within the hospital (and therefore via an outpatient supply form), there may be situations where it is necessary for the item to be supplied within the community. In these situations, it is necessary for the prescriber to prescribe the item(s) via an NHS prescription form (i.e. via an FP10HNC or equivalent).

The dispensing procedure for hospital supply

As with the supply of medication against an NHS prescription form (see Chapter 3) the supply of medication within a hospital setting can be divided into a number of distinct sections.

Upon receipt of an order for medication within a hospital, the following procedure should be followed:

1. Identify the order type.
2. Check that all necessary information is present on the order.
3. If appropriate, perform a clinical check on the prescription.
4. Dispense and label the item(s) as necessary.
5. Check the item(s) dispensed is/are correct and labelled appropriately; ideally this check would be performed by a colleague (i.e. an independent check) but, when working alone, the pharmacist will need to check the item(s) him- or herself.
6. If appropriate, pass the item(s) to the patient and counsel the patient in the use of the medication.

KeyPoints

The dispensing procedure for hospital orders:

1. Identify the order type.
2. Check all necessary information is present on the order.
3. If appropriate, perform a clinical check on the prescription.
4. Dispense and label the item(s) as necessary.
5. Check the item(s) dispensed is/are correct and labelled appropriately.
6. If appropriate, pass the item(s) to the patient and counsel the patient in the use of the medication.

Worked examples

This chapter contains worked examples and self-assessment questions using a variety of different hospital medication orders (inpatient orders, TTOs and outpatient prescriptions) for dispensing in a hospital pharmacy. Although a number of different examples are used in this section, all orders can be addressed by using a standard systematic approach.

Example 4.1

This example is similar to Example 3.1 in Chapter 3, the difference being that, instead of the item being prescribed by a dentist on an NHS prescription form, it has been prescribed as a TTO for a patient who is being discharged from a hospital ward. Note the differences between the dispensing process for this example and Example 3.1.

You receive the TTO shown in Figure 4.2 in your pharmacy.

1. Identity of order
Hospital TTO (TTA) discharge prescription.

2. Prescriber
Doctor (hospital doctor).

3. Legally written?
Yes.

4. Clinical check (complete Table 4.1)

Table 4.1

Drug	Indications	Dose check	Reference
Co-amoxiclav	Infections caused by β-lactamase-producing strains	Expressed as amoxicillin 250 mg every 8 h, dose doubled in severe infections	*British National Formulary*, 56th edn, section 5.1.1

5. Interactions
There is only one drug on the TTO. However, it would also be advisable for the pharmacist or pharmacy technician to check the patient's inpatient chart for any concurrent medication that could cause an interaction. Although a patient would need to continue to take all prescribed medication on discharge, he or she may already have enough of some medication, so that medication may not appear on the TTO. This situation is especially likely to occur if the patient is part of a POD scheme.

6. Suitability for patient
Item prescribed is safe and suitable for a patient of this age and the dose ordered on the prescription is within the recommended dose limits.

Figure 4.1 Framework for systematic dispensing/supply of hospital prescriptions or medication orders.

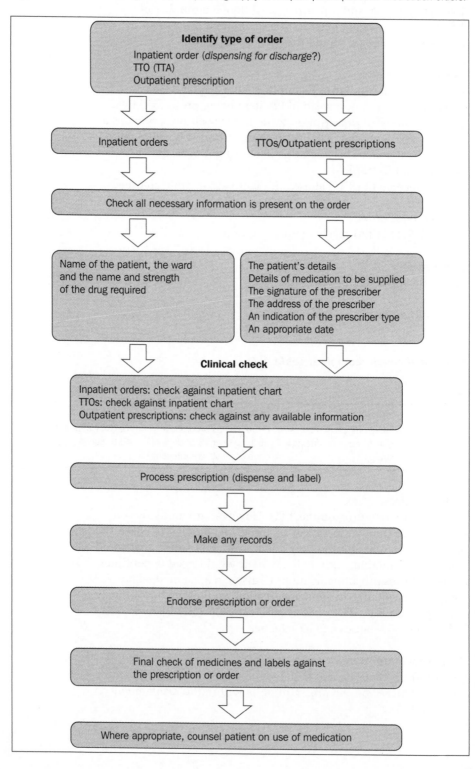

Figure 4.2

ANYWHERE HOSPITAL

ANYWHERE

DISCHARGE MEDICATION

Patient's Name: Harry Baker

Patient's address: 54 Somerset Place

Ward: Ward 9

Details of in-patient medication required:

Drug	Dosage and Instructions	Pharmacy
Co-amoxiclav	250/125 tds 7/7	

Prescriber: Julie Timmins   **Bleep:** 3474

7. Records to be made (including copies of the record[s])
None.

8. Process prescription (including example of label[s])
- The quantity of medication to be supplied has been stated. For most medication supplied on a TTO, the quantity supplied would be based on hospital policy (usually around 14 days). However, as this item is an antibiotic, the prescriber has indicated that enough for the entire course (i.e. 1 week) should be supplied.
- Check appendix 9 of the *British National Formulary* for supplementary labelling requirements:
  - Co-amoxiclav: *British National Formulary* label number 9. (Take at regular intervals. Complete the prescribed course unless otherwise directed.)
- It is usual for labels for antibiotics supplied by hospitals to indicate the spacing of doses (i.e. every 8 h), rather than the frequency of administration (i.e. three times a day). If this item were on a prescription form in the community (FP10 or equivalent), then the directions on the label would be the same as those on the prescription.

- Select co-amoxiclav tablets from shelf, remembering to check expiry date.
- Perform final check of item, label and prescription.
- Pack in a suitable bag ready to give to patient/patient's representative.

Labels (we have assumed that the name and address of the pharmacy and the words 'Keep out of the reach and sight of children' are pre-printed on the label) (Figure 4.3).

Figure 4.3

Co-amoxiclav 250/125 Tablets	21
Take ONE tablet every EIGHT hours.	
Take at regular intervals. Complete the prescribed course unless otherwise directed.	
Mr Harry Baker	Date of dispensing

9. Endorse prescription

Endorse the pharmacy box on the TTO with the details of the medication supplied and initials of the pharmacist and pharmacy technician(s) involved in the dispensing process.

10. Destination of paperwork

Either the original or a copy of the TTO is kept with the patient's hospital notes at the hospital. In addition, a copy may be supplied to the patient's GP.

11. Identity check/counselling

The medication needs to be given to the patient. In most cases, either the patient comes down to the pharmacy to collect his medication as he is leaving the hospital or the medication is sent to the patient's ward and given to him by the ward pharmacist or a member of the nursing staff on discharge. In both cases, the following information needs to be given to the patient or his representative.

- Check patient's name and address.
- Reinforce the dosage; take the medication at regular intervals (8 hourly) and complete the prescribed course.
- Draw patient's attention to the patient information leaflet (PIL) and ask if he has any questions.

Example 4.2

You receive the outpatient prescription in Figure 4.4 in your hospital pharmacy.

1. Identity of order

Outpatient prescription.

Figure 4.4

```
ANYWHERE HOSPITAL
ANYWHERE

        OUT-PATIENT PRESCRIPTION

Patient's Name:   Simon BELL
Patient's address: 45 Dingle Lane, Anytown

Details of medication required:

Dovonex Cream
Mitte 1 X OP
Sig apply tds



Prescriber: June Littlewood
```

2. Prescriber
Doctor (hospital consultant).

3. Legally written?
Yes.

4. Clinical check (complete Table 4.2)

Table 4.2

Drug	Indications	Dose check	Reference
Calcipotriol	Plaque psoriasis	Apply once or twice daily	British National Formulary, 56th edn, section 13.5

There is only one item on the prescription form. However, it would also be advisable for the pharmacist or pharmacy technician to check, where possible, the PMR for any concurrent medication that could cause an interaction.

5. Suitability for patient
Item prescribed is safe and suitable for a patient of this age but the instructions for use on the prescription (i.e. to apply three times a day) are not within the recommended limits. Contact prescriber to check her intentions and arrange for the prescription to be changed to a more acceptable frequency (e.g. once or twice a day).

6. Records to be made (including copies of the record[s])
Make a note of the intervention on a clinical intervention form.

7. Process prescription (including example of label[s])
- Prepare label for product.
- Check appendix 9 of the *British National Formulary* for supplementary labelling requirements (there are none).
- Remember to add pharmaceutical cautions to label (for external use only).
- Select tube of Dovonex cream from shelf, remembering to check the expiry date; as '1 × op' has been requested, the smallest pack size (60 g) should be supplied.
- Label the primary container (i.e. the tube not the box).
- Perform final check of item, label and prescription form.
- Pack in a suitable bag ready to give to patient/patient's representative.

Labels (we have assumed that the name and address of the pharmacy and the words 'Keep out of the reach and sight of children' are pre-printed on the label) (Figure 4.5).

Figure 4.5

Dovonex Cream	60 g
Apply TWICE a day.	
For External Use Only.	
Mr Simon Bell	Date of dispensing

8. Endorse prescription
Endorse the outpatient prescription with the details of the medication supplied and initials of the pharmacist and pharmacy technician(s) involved in the dispensing process.

9. Destination of paperwork
File the prescription within the hospital according to local procedures.

10. Identity check/counselling
- Check patient's name and address.
- Advise patient of change in directions of use without alarming him.
- Reinforce new dosage instructions and that it is for external use only.
- Draw patient's attention to the PIL and ask if he has any questions.

Self-assessment

The following section of questions contains examples of prescriptions that may be encountered in a hospital pharmacy. In each case, complete the sections to guide you through the dispensing process (note that compared with the dispensing of NHS prescriptions, there is no need to check whether the item[s] are allowable on the NHS – they would be unless the items were prescribed on a hospital NHS prescription form as the prescription would be intended to be dispensed within the community):

1. identity of order
2. prescriber
3. legally written?
4. clinical check (complete Table 4.3)
5. interactions
6. suitability for patient
7. records to be made (including copies of the record[s])
8. process prescription (including example of label[s])
9. endorse prescription
10. destination of paperwork
11. identity check/counselling.

Table 4.3

Drug	Indications	Dose check	Reference

Question 1

You are the ward pharmacist for Ward 26 (a medical ward) and are asked by the nursing staff to order from the hospital pharmacy the antibiotics for Mary Smith that have just been written on the patient's drug chart by the doctor (Ward 26 does not hold ciprofloxacin tablets as ward stock).

The chart looks like Figure 4.6 (only the part of the page with entries on has been shown here).

Using the sections indicated above, summarise all stages of the dispensing process for this item (the ciprofloxacin).

Question 2

You receive the outpatient prescription shown in Figure 4.7 in your pharmacy.

Using the sections indicated above, summarise all stages of the dispensing process for this prescription form.

Question 3

You receive the TTO shown in Figure 4.8 in your pharmacy.

Using the sections indicated above, summarise all stages of the dispensing process for this prescription form.

Figure 4.6

Surname:	Smith		Ward:		26					
First Name:	Mary Ann		Consultant:		Smith					
Patient Number:	123456		Date of Birth:		18/07/69					
Regular medication		Date:	1/9	2/9	3/9					
Drug name:	Frequency	(08.00)	CL	CL						
Digoxin 250 mcg	Daily	10.00								
Signature:	Route	12.00								
A Hardy	Oral	14.00								
Pharmacy	Date	18.00								
T Jones (Pts own)	01/09/08	22.00								
Drug name:	Frequency	08.00								
Ciprofloxacin 250 mg	BD	(10.00)	x ——							
Signature:	Route	12.00								
A Hardy	Oral	14.00								
Pharmacy	Date	18.00								
	02/09/08	(22.00)	x							x

Figure 4.7

ANYWHERE HOSPITAL
ANYWHERE

OUTPATIENT PRESCRIPTION

Patient's Name: Anthony GREENWOOD
Patient's address: 4 The Chase, Anytown

Details of medication required:

Ketorolac 10 mg tablets
Mitte 20
Sig i 4–6 hourly mdu

Prescriber: John Donovan

Figure 4.8

ANYWHERE HOSPITAL

ANYWHERE

DISCHARGE MEDICATION

Patient's Name: Bob Cooper

Patient's address: 102 Wheelwright Avenue

Ward: Ward 15

Details of medication required:

Drug	Dosage and Instructions	Pharmacy
Amlodipine	5 mg OD	

Prescriber: Manjit Kaur   Bleep: 5489

Summary

This chapter has covered the key points with which it is necessary to be familiar in order to supply medication to patients within a hospital setting. It is important that pharmacists and pharmacy technicians are familiar with the different types of hospital supply (inpatient orders, TTOs and outpatient prescriptions) and the new variants of these (e.g. dispensing for discharge schemes or POD schemes).

Finally, it should be remembered that, in many cases, different rules apply to what may be supplied via an inpatient medication order or TTO/outpatient prescription compared with NHS supply in primary care. The main difference between these types of supply and NHS supply (see Chapters 2 and 3) is that the *Drug Tariff* rules do not apply.

chapter 5
Non-NHS supply

Overview

Upon completion of this chapter, you should be able to:
- understand the general dispensing procedure for non-NHS (private) prescriptions in the community
- understand the general dispensing procedure for requisitions in the community
- complete a number of worked examples and self-assessment questions containing non-NHS (private) prescriptions
- complete a number of worked examples and self-assessment questions containing requisitions.

Introduction and overview

This chapter summarises all types of supply that are outside normal NHS supply. The following topics are covered:
- the supply of medication via non-NHS (private) prescriptions
- the supply of medicinal products via written or oral requisitions.

The private supply of medication to patients within hospitals is similar to NHS hospital supply and was covered in Chapter 4.

Non-NHS (private) prescription supply

Many patients who require medication are supplied via the NHS either within the community (see Chapters 2 and 3) or in a hospital setting (see Chapter 4). However, an alternative to this would be to supply medication privately (i.e. outside the NHS). In these cases, the patient is charged the cost of the item(s) plus a mark-up, and a fee levied by the pharmacist as payment for dispensing the item(s).

The dispensing procedure for non-NHS (private) prescriptions is similar to the dispensing procedure followed with NHS prescriptions (see Chapter 3). The main differences are that, in most cases, an entry detailing the supply always needs to be made in the prescription-only medicines register and that the pharmacist or pharmacy technician does not need to check that the item is allowed on the NHS. In summary, the procedure to be followed is as follows:

1. Check the legality of the non-NHS (private) prescription form.
2. Identify the prescriber.
3. Perform a clinical check on the prescription.

KeyPoints

KeyPoint

4. Dispense and label the item(s), including making a prescription-only medicines register entry.
5. Check the item(s) dispensed is/are correct and labelled appropriately; ideally this check would be performed by a colleague (i.e. an independent check) but, when working alone, the pharmacist needs to check the item(s) him- or herself.
6. Pass the item(s) to the patient and counsel the patient in the use of the medication.
7. Process the prescription form.

Repeatable non-NHS (private) prescription forms

Unlike NHS prescription forms, non-NHS (private) prescription forms may be repeatable (except in the case of non-NHS (private) prescription forms for Schedule 2 and 3 controlled drugs – see Chapter 6). In this situation, the prescriber annotates the prescription form to indicate that the prescription may be dispensed more than once.

The prescription-only medicines register

It is a legal requirement to record the sale or supply of all prescription-only medicines (POMs) not supplied via the NHS (i.e. on an NHS prescription form) in the community unless:

- a separate record of the sale or supply is made in accordance with the Misuse of Drugs Regulations 2001
- a sale is by way of wholesale dealing and a copy of the order or invoice relating thereto is retained by the owner of the retail pharmacy business
- the supply is for an oral contraceptive.

However, in all cases it is still considered good practice to make an entry (as it would be for non-NHS [private] prescriptions or wholesale dealing of non-POMs, i.e. for general sale list or pharmacy [GSL/P] medicines).

Records of medication supply are made in the POM register in the following instances:

- medication supply via a non-NHS (private) prescription

- supply of medication via a written requisition
- supply of medication in response to an oral requisition
- emergency supply of medication at the request of a practitioner (see Chapter 7)
- emergency supply of POM at the request of a patient (see Chapter 7).

Figure 5.1 shows a standard POM register page.

Figure 5.1 An example of a standard prescription-only medicines register page.

Reference number	Details		Cost

The detail of what needs to be recorded in each of the sections in Figure 5.1 in various different circumstances can be found in the relevant sections of this book. The POM register must be kept at the premises to which it relates during its period of use and for 2 years after the last entry. Each entry has a unique reference number, usually made up of the page number and entry number on that page (e.g. on page 12, the first entry is '12.1', the second '12.2', etc).

Written requisitions

In addition to the supply of medication on the NHS via individual prescription forms (see Chapters 2 and 3) or hospital order (see Chapter 4), and the supply of medication via non-NHS (private) prescription forms, it is also necessary to become familiar with other forms of supply. These are where practitioners or other authorised individuals require a medicinal product for use during the course of their practice or business. This may not, at this stage, be for a named patient. This would include, for example, where a GP requests something for use during home visits or an optician requests a medicinal item for use during eye examinations.

Supplies of medication normally take place via a written requisition (colloquially known as a 'signed order', although the term is somewhat misleading because most written requisitions do not actually need to be signed). In addition, it is also permissible for some individuals to request medication supply verbally.

> ## KeyPoints
>
> Records of medication supply are made in the prescription-only medicine (POM) register in the following instances:
> - medication supply via a non-NHS (private) prescription
> - supply of medication via a written requisition
> - supply of medication in response to an oral requisition
> - emergency supply of medication at the request of a practitioner
> - emergency supply of POM at the request of a patient.
>
> The POM register must be kept at the premises to which it relates during its period of use and for 2 years after the last entry.

General requisition layout

Except where detailed in the following section, for a written requisition for POMs there are no legally defined details as to the content required. However, it would be reasonable to expect the requisition to provide enough information to make a POM register entry. We suggest, therefore, that the following list would be a good starting point:

- Details of preparation (sufficient to be clear as to which product has been requested, i.e. name, quantity, form and strength as appropriate)
- Name and address, trade business or profession of the person to whom the medicine is supplied
- The purpose for which the medicine is supplied
- Signature of prescriber.

It is worth noting at this point that requisitions for controlled drugs have additional requirements, which are discussed in Chapter 6.

When supplying medication via a written requisition, it should be noted that only complete packs (including any patient information leaflets – PILs) can be supplied. As the medication is usually not for a specific patient (at the point at which the requisition is made), there is no need to label the medication. If the medication were for a specific patient, it would be usual to issue a patient-specific prescription form (either an NHS or non-NHS [private] prescription form).

It is good practice to make an entry in the POM register at the time of supply; it is only a good practice requirement because the requisition is retained within the pharmacy for 2 years from the date of supply (the exception to this is for Schedules 2 and 3 controlled drugs where a photocopy is kept). However, if the request was an oral one (see below), the POM register entry would be a legal requirement (as there is no paper requisition detailing the sale to keep for 2 years).

For completeness, it is also worth mentioning that it is not a legal requirement to make an entry in the POM register if a separate record of the sale or supply is made in the controlled drugs register. However, it is still good practice to make an entry in the POM register.

The sale or supply of medication may be made to a number of individuals including:

- appropriate nurse prescribers
- chiropodists/podiatrists
- hospitals or health centres
- midwives
- occupational health schemes
- opticians
- other pharmacies

- owners and masters of ships including foreign vessels
- practitioners
- other individuals, exempted people and organisations.

Full details on these individuals and what they may be supplied with can be found in *Applied Pharmaceutical Practice* (Langley and Belcher, 2008) or the current edition of *Medicines, Ethics and Practice – A guide for pharmacists and pharmacy technicians* (see Bibliography).

Oral requests for medicine supply by practitioners

In addition to written requests by a variety of healthcare practitioners and other authorised individuals, some requests for the supply of medication do not have to be written down (i.e. via a written requisition). These are termed 'oral requisitions'.

Oral requests may be made by any of the individuals who may request medication via written requisitions, except in the following cases:

- the supply of POMs to an optician
- the supply of any Schedule 2 or 3 controlled drugs, including the supply of diamorphine, morphine, pentazocine and pethidine to midwives, which requires a midwives' supply order.

Remember that, for oral requests, there is no written request for the supply and so it is a legal requirement that an entry be made in the POM register.

The dispensing procedure for non-NHS prescriptions

The dispensing procedure to be followed upon receipt of a non-NHS (private) prescription is similar to that of an NHS prescription (see Chapter 3). The main difference is that the pharmacist or pharmacy technician does not have to check whether the item is allowable on the NHS (as the prescribing is taking place outside the NHS).

Therefore, in summary, the following procedure should be followed:

1. Check the legality of the non-NHS (private) prescription.
2. Identify the prescriber.
3. Perform a clinical check on the prescription.
4. Dispense and label the item(s).

KeyPoints

The dispensing procedure for non-NHS (private) prescriptions:

1. Check the legality of the non-NHS (private) prescription form.
2. Identify the prescriber.
3. Perform a clinical check on the prescription.
4. Dispense and label the item(s).
5. Check the item(s) dispensed is/are correct and labelled appropriately.
6. Pass the item(s) to the patient and counsel the patient in the use of the medication.
7. Process the prescription form.

5. Check that the item(s) dispensed is/are correct and labelled appropriately; ideally this check would be performed by a colleague (i.e. an independent check) but, when working alone, the pharmacist will need to check the item(s) him- or herself.
6. Pass the item(s) to the patient and counsel the patient in the use of the medication.
7. Process the prescription form.

Worked examples

Although a number of different examples are used in this section, all prescription forms can be addressed by using a standard systematic approach (see Chapter 3).

Example 5.1

You receive the prescription shown in Figure 5.2 in your pharmacy.

Figure 5.2

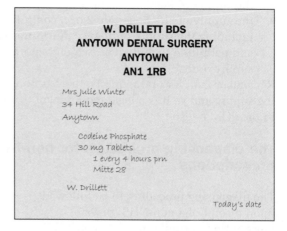

W. DRILLETT BDS
ANYTOWN DENTAL SURGERY
ANYTOWN
AN1 1RB

Mrs Julie Winter
34 Hill Road
Anytown

Codeine Phosphate
30 mg Tablets
1 every 4 hours prn
Mitte 28

W. Drillett

Today's date

1. Identity of order
Private prescription.

2. Prescriber
Dentist (the prescriber is a local dentist).

3. Legally written?
Yes. The item (codeine phosphate tablets) is not listed within the *Dental Practitioners' Formulary*; however, as this is a private prescription form, the dentist is not limited to prescribing from within this list.

Nevertheless, you should still ensure that the dentist is prescribing within his or her area of competence. As this prescription form is for an analgesic, this prescribing is likely to be within the dentist's area of competence and so it would be acceptable to make the supply without any further information.

4. Clinical check (complete Table 5.1)

Table 5.1

Drug	Indications	Dose check	Reference
Codeine phosphate	Mild-to-moderate pain	30–60 mg every 4 h when necessary. Max. 240 mg daily	*British National Formulary* 56th edn, section 4.7.2

5. Interactions

There is only one item on the prescription form. However, it would also be advisable for the pharmacist or pharmacy technician to check the patient's medication record (PMR) for any concurrent medication that could cause an interaction.

6. Suitability for patient

The item prescribed is safe and suitable for an adult patient and the dose ordered on the prescription is within the recommended dose limits.

7. Records to be made (including copies of the record[s])

A POM register entry is required (Figure 5.3).

Figure 5.3

Reference number	Details	Cost
5.01 Date of supply	Mrs Julie Winter 34 Hill Road Anytown Codeine Phosphate Tablets 30 mg 1 every 4 hours prn (28 tablets) W. Drillett BDS Anytown Dental Surgery Anytown AN1 1RB Date on prescription: Today's	Cost + 50% + Dispensing fee + Container fee

8. Process prescription (including example of label[s])

- Prepare a label.
- Check appendix 9 of the *British National Formulary* for supplementary labelling requirements:
  - Codeine phosphate: *British National Formulary* label number 2 (Warning: may cause drowsiness. If affected do not drive or operate machinery. Avoid alcoholic drink.)
- Select codeine phosphate tablets from shelf, remembering to check expiry date.
- Perform final check of item, label and prescription.
- Pack in a suitable bag ready to give to patient/patient's representative.

Labels (we have assumed that the name and address of the pharmacy and the words 'Keep out of the reach and sight of children' are pre-printed on the label) (Figure 5.4).

Figure 5.4

Codeine Phosphate 30 mg Tablets	28
Take ONE tablet every four hours when required.	
Warning. May cause drowsiness.	
If affected do not drive or operate machinery.	
Avoid alcoholic drink.	
Mrs Julie Winter	Date of dispensing

9. Endorse prescription

Stamp with pharmacy stamp to indicate completion and annotate stamp with the POM register entry number (5.01).

10. Destination of paperwork

Retain prescription in pharmacy for 2 years.

11. Identity check/counselling

- Check patient's name and address.
- Reinforce the dosage instructions.
- Advise the patient that the tablets may cause drowsiness and, if affected, don't drive or operate machinery.
- Draw patient's attention to the PIL and ask if she has any questions.

Example 5.2

You receive the prescription shown in Figure 5.5 in your pharmacy.

1. Identity of order

Private prescription.

2. Prescriber

Doctor (the prescriber is a local doctor).

Figure 5.5

```
ANYWHERE HEALTH CENTRE
        ANYTOWN
        AN1 1RB


Mrs Sheila Smith

   Trimethoprim Tablets
      200mg bd 7/7
   Bendroflumethiazide Tablets
      2.5mg od. Mitte 28.

  R U Better
                        Today's date
```

3. Legally written?

No. The doctor has failed to add the patient's address to the prescription and (although we may know from local knowledge) there is also no indication of type of prescriber on the prescription. This is usually indicated by the addition of qualifications to the prescription.

Return the prescription to the prescriber for addition of address and indication of authority to prescribe (e.g. 'MB ChB') before dispensing.

4. Clinical check (complete Table 5.2)

Table 5.2

Drug	Indications	Dose check	Reference
Trimethoprim	Urinary tract infections, acute and chronic bronchitis	200 mg every 12 h	British National Formulary, 56th edn, section 5.1.8
Bendroflumethiazide	Hypertension	2.5 mg in the morning	British National Formulary, 56th edn, section 2.2.1

5. Interactions

There is no interaction between trimethoprim and bendroflumethiazide. However, it would also be advisable for the pharmacist or pharmacy technician to check the PMR for any concurrent medication that could cause an interaction.

6. Suitability for patient

The items prescribed are safe and suitable for an adult patient and the doses ordered on the prescription are within the recommended dose limits.

7. Records to be made (including copies of the record[s])

A POM register entry is required (Figure 5.6).

Figure 5.6

Reference number	Details	Cost

5.02
 	
Date of supply
	Mrs Sheila Smith
	
	14 Boot Lane, Anytown
	
	(1) Trimethoprim Tablets
	      200mg bd 7/7.
	(2) Bendroflumethiazide Tablets
	      2.5mg od. Mitte 28.
	
	R U Better MB ChB
	Anytown Health Centre
	Anytown
	
	Date on prescription: Today's
	
	Prescriber contacted to add patient's address and his qualifications.
		Cost
		+
		50%
		+
		Dispensing fee
		+
		Container fee

A note of the intervention on a clinical intervention form is not necessary in this case because the intervention has been recorded in the POM register.

8. Process prescription (including example of label[s])
- Prepare label for each product.
- Check appendix 9 of the *British National Formulary* for supplementary labelling requirements:
  - Trimethoprim: *British National Formulary* label number 9 (Take at regular intervals. Complete the prescribed course unless otherwise directed.)
    Bendroflumethiazide: no additional labels.
- Select tablets from shelf, remembering to check expiry dates.
- Perform final check of items, labels and prescription form.
- Pack in a suitable bag ready to give to patient/patient's representative.

Labels (we have assumed that the name and address of the pharmacy and the words 'Keep out of the reach and sight of children' are pre-printed on the label) (Figure 5.7).

9. Endorse prescription
Stamp with pharmacy stamp to indicate completion and annotate stamp with the POM register entry numbers (5.02[1] and 5.02[2]).

10. Destination of paperwork
Retain prescription in pharmacy for 2 years.

Figure 5.7

Trimethoprim 200 mg Tablets	14
Take ONE tablet TWICE a day.	
Take at regular intervals.	
Complete the prescribed course	
unless otherwise directed.	
Mrs Sheila Smith	Date of dispensing

Bendroflumethiazide 2.5 mg Tablets	28
Take ONE tablet daily.	
Mrs Sheila Smith	Date of dispensing

11. Identity check/counselling

- Check patient's name and address.
- Reinforce the dosage instructions.
- Stress importance of taking trimethoprim regularly (every 12 hours) and completing the course.
- Advise that bendroflumethiazide should normally be taken in the morning because she may need to go to toilet more frequently within 2 hours of taking the medication.
- Draw patient's attention to the PIL and ask if she has any questions.

Self-assessment

This section of questions contains examples of non-NHS (private) prescription forms and requisitions for dispensing within a community pharmacy. In each case, complete the sections to guide you through the dispensing process.

Private (non-NHS) prescriptions

Note that compared with the dispensing of NHS prescriptions, there is no need to check whether the item(s) is/are allowable on the NHS:

1. identity of order
2. prescriber
3. legally written?
4. clinical check (complete Table 5.3)

Table 5.3

Drug	Indications	Dose check	Reference

5. interactions
6. suitability for patient
7. records to be made (including copies of the record[s])
8. process prescription (including example of label[s])
9. endorse prescription
10. destination of paperwork
11. identity check/counselling.

Question 1

You receive the prescription shown in Figure 5.8 in your pharmacy.

Using the sections indicated above, summarise all stages of the dispensing process for this prescription form.

Figure 5.8

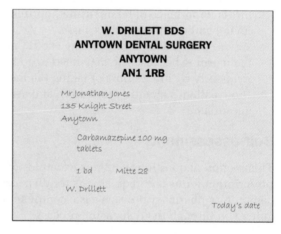

Question 2

You receive the prescription shown in Figure 5.9 in your pharmacy.

Using the sections indicated above, summarise all stages of the dispensing process for this prescription form.

Figure 5.9

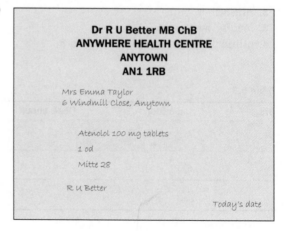

Requisitions

Note that compared with the dispensing of NHS prescriptions and
non-NHS (private) prescriptions, there is no need to perform a
clinical check, check for interactions, check the suitability of the
item(s) for the patient or check whether the item(s) are allowable
on the NHS because (except for some patient-specific written
requests from optometrists) there is no patient:

1. identity of order
2. requisitioner
3. legally written?
4. records to be made (including copies of the record[s])
5. process requisition
6. endorse requisition
7. destination of paperwork
8. identity check/counselling.

Although a number of different examples are used in this section,
from a variety of different prescribers, all prescription forms can
be addressed by using a standard systematic approach (see
Chapter 3).

Question 3

You receive the requisition shown in Figure 5.10 in your
pharmacy.

Using the sections indicated above, summarise all stages of the
dispensing process for this written requisition.

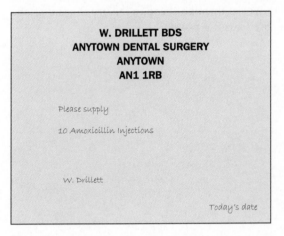

Figure 5.10.

W. DRILLETT BDS
ANYTOWN DENTAL SURGERY
ANYTOWN
AN1 1RB

Please supply

10 Amoxicillin Injections

W. Drillett

Today's date

Question 4

You receive the requisition in Figure 5.11 in your pharmacy.

Using the sections indicated above, summarise all stages of the
dispensing process for this written requisition.

Figure 5.11

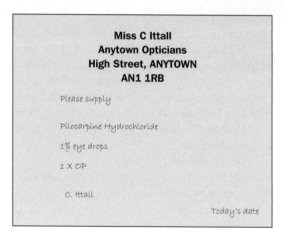

Miss C Ittall
Anytown Opticians
High Street, ANYTOWN
AN1 1RB

Please supply

Pilocarpine Hydrochloride

1% eye drops

1 X OP

C. Ittall

Today's date

Summary

This chapter has covered the key points with which it is necessary to be familiar in order to supply medication via non-NHS prescription forms (private prescriptions) and via both written and oral requisitions. This has included details on who may requisition medicines and the restrictions placed on different healthcare practitioners.

Worked examples and self-assessment questions have been provided and it is suggested that the student pharmacist or pharmacy technician works through these to ensure that he or she is familiar with the key learning points.

chapter 6
Controlled drugs

Overview

Upon completion of this chapter, you should be able to:

- understand how controlled drugs are classified within pharmacy
- list authorised prescribers of controlled drugs
- be familiar with the different prescription requirements for controlled drugs
- understand the purpose of specific non-NHS (private) prescription forms for controlled drugs
- be familiar with the dispensing procedure for controlled drugs, including the use of addict (instalment) prescriptions
- understand the procedures involved with the supply of controlled drugs via written requisitions
- summarise the legislation relating to the record keeping, storage and destruction of controlled drugs
- complete a number of worked examples and self-assessment questions of prescriptions containing controlled drugs and the dispensing process.

Introduction and overview

Some drugs have increased measures placed upon them relating to possession and supply. Within pharmacy, these are termed 'controlled drugs' or more commonly CDs. This chapter highlights the key parts of the Misuse of Drugs Act 1971 and Misuse of Drugs Regulations 2001 (and subsequent amendments) that are relevant to current pharmaceutical practice. However, this is an area that at the time of writing is going through some key changes. Therefore, in a similar way to developments within clinical practice, it is the responsibility of the individual pharmacist and pharmacy technician to ensure that they are up to date with any changes to the legislation covering controlled drugs.

Classification of controlled drugs

The Misuse of Drugs Act 1971 classifies controlled drugs into three classes: A, B and C. These classes reflect the level of harm that the drug may do to individuals (with class A being the highest level) but no classification is linked to whether the drug is used within medicine. The higher the class, the higher the penalties applied for possession and supply (i.e. dealing). In addition, drugs may move between classes as a result of changes in the legislation.

KeyPoints

For day-to-day use in pharmacy, the classification of controlled drugs into different schedules is used. The schedules reflect better the use of the individual controlled drugs within medicine and are more useful. These schedules are set out in the Misuse of Drugs Regulations.

The easiest way to identify which schedule of the Misuse of Drugs Act classifies a drug is to refer to a current edition of *Medicines, Ethics and Practice: A guide for pharmacists and pharmacy technicians* (see Bibliography). Within the 'Alphabetical list of medicines for human use' of this book, the list uses the following abbreviations to indicate the schedule(s) that applies(y) to the drug:

- CD POM: Schedule 2
- CD No Reg POM: Schedule 3
- CD Benz POM: Schedule 4, Part I
- CD Anab POM: Schedule 4, Part II
- CD Inv POM or CD Inv P: Schedule 5.

Pharmacists and pharmacy technicians need to take care when using this list because one drug may appear in more than one schedule, depending on the strength of the drug within a particular preparation. For example, morphine sulphate is a Schedule 2 controlled drug when it is in an injectable form. However, within Kaolin and Morphine Mixture BP, the morphine is classified as a Schedule 5 drug because of the low concentration of morphine within the preparation.

Prescribers of controlled drugs

Until recently, the numbers of individuals who could prescribe controlled drugs were fairly limited. However, with the onset of both supplementary and independent prescribing, the numbers of individuals who may prescribe controlled drugs have increased.

Currently, the following individuals may prescribe controlled drugs:

- Doctors, dentists and vets may prescribe all Schedules 2–5 controlled drugs. Doctors can only prescribe diamorphine, dipipanone or cocaine for the treatment of addiction with a licence from the Home Office (although they can prescribe these drugs for any other medical purpose).
- Nurses who are independent non-medical prescribers (formerly extended formulary nurse prescribers) may prescribe certain controlled drugs for certain medical

conditions. These drugs and the conditions within which they may be prescribed can be found in *Applied Pharmaceutical Practice* (Langley and Belcher, 2008) or the current edition of *Medicines, Ethics and Practice: A guide for pharmacists and pharmacy technicians.*

- Some controlled drugs can be supplied or administered via patient group directions.
- Supplementary prescribers can prescribe some controlled drugs via clinical management plans.
- Midwives can possess, supply and administer diamorphine, morphine, pethidine and pentazocine, provided that it is in the course of their professional midwifery practice.

Prescription requirements

Prescriptions for Schedules 2 and 3 controlled drugs have additional requirements, above and beyond what would normally be required on a prescription for it to be legally dispensed.

Pharmacists CAN supply Schedules 2 and 3 controlled drugs (except temazepam) against some prescriptions that have a minor technical error but where the prescriber's intention is clear. The only errors that pharmacists can currently amend are minor typographical errors or spelling mistakes, or where the total quantity of the preparation of the controlled drug or the number of dosage units, as the case may be, is specified in either words or figures but not both (i.e. they can add the words *or* the figures to the controlled drug prescription if they have been omitted).

The pharmacist amends the prescription in ink or otherwise indelibly to correct the minor typographical errors or spelling mistakes, or adds the total quantity of drug or number of dosage units in either words *or* figures so that the prescription complies with the controlled drug prescription requirements. In addition the pharmacist should mark the prescription so that the

KeyPoints

Prescriptions for Schedules 2 and 3 controlled drugs must*:
- be signed by the prescriber
- be dated
- be written so as to be indelible
- specify the address of the prescriber
- for a private prescription (including temazepam) be written on an FP10PCD
- specify the dose to be taken
- specify the form of the preparation
- specify, where appropriate, the strength of the preparation
- specify either the total quantity (in both words and figures) of the preparation or (in both words and figures) the number of dosage units
- have written on them, if for dental treatment, the words 'for dental treatment only'
- specify the name and address of the patient.

* Note that some of the requirements listed above do not apply to prescriptions for the drug temazepam.

Recent key changes to prescription requirements applicable to controlled drugs are as follows:
- Prescriptions no longer need to be in the prescriber's own handwriting.
- The validity of controlled drug prescriptions has been reduced from 13 weeks to 28 days.
- It is good practice for prescribers to limit their prescribing to 30 days' supply.
- It is good practice for prescribers not to prescribe controlled drugs for themselves or close family members unless in an emergency.

amendment made is attributable to them (e.g. annotate the amendment with the pharmacist's signature/initials and registration number).

Non-NHS (private) prescription forms for controlled drugs

Recent changes to the legislation have meant that private (non-NHS) prescription forms for Schedule 2 and 3 controlled drugs for dispensing within the community (for human use) must be on a specific form, known as an FP10PCD (England), PPCD(1) (Scotland) or WP10PCD/WP10PCDSS (Wales). Although resembling an NHS prescription, the FP10PCD (and equivalents) is a private prescription. After dispensing, these private prescription forms are sent to the Prescription Pricing Division (PPD or equivalent) at the end of the month (in a similar way to NHS prescriptions) for monitoring purposes. It should also be noted that private prescriptions for Schedules 2 and 3 controlled drugs are not repeatable.

The dispensing procedure

KeyPoints

When dispensing a prescription for a controlled drug, pharmacists and pharmacy technicians need to take the following points into consideration: a prescription for a controlled drug must not be dispensed:

- unless it complies with the requirements
- if the prescriber's address given on the prescription is not within the UK (for Schedules 2 and 3 controlled drugs)
- unless the prescriber's signature is genuine
- before the date specified on the prescription
- more than 28 days after the date on the prescription (or specified start date).

In addition:

- The date of each supply must be marked on the prescription.
- Repeats of Schedules 2 and 3 drugs are not allowed, but instalments are.
- For private prescriptions, a prescription-only medicines register entry is not legally required if a controlled drugs register entry is made, but it is still good practice to do so.
- Emergency supplies of Schedules 2 and 3 controlled drugs are not allowed except phenobarbital for the treatment of epilepsy.

Collection of prescriptions for controlled drugs

Recent changes to the regulations have meant that additional steps need to be taken by pharmacists and pharmacy technicians when handing out medication containing controlled drugs. These additional requirements can be summarised as follows:

- Pharmacists must ascertain whether the person collecting a Schedule 2 controlled drug is the patient, the patient's representative or a healthcare professional acting in his or her capacity as such.

- If the person collecting the Schedule 2 controlled drug is a healthcare professional acting in a professional capacity on behalf of the patient, the pharmacist must obtain the name and address of the healthcare professional and, unless already acquainted with that person, he or she should request evidence of that person's identity (however, even if identification is not provided, the pharmacist may still supply the controlled drug).
- Pharmacists are expected to ask for identification upon collection of Schedule 2 controlled drug and to obtain a signature on the back of prescription.
- Pharmacists have the discretion not to ask for identification but this must be recorded in the controlled drug register.
- The collection of Schedule 3 controlled drugs does not require identification, but the collector is still expected to sign the back of the prescription.

Addict (instalment) prescriptions for controlled drugs

The treatment of addiction to certain drugs may use substitution therapy. This is where the drug that the patient is addicted to is substituted for another drug which may be prescribed on a prescription form. Drugs allowed as substitutes are (most commonly) methadone, buprenorphine, dextromoramide, morphine and pethidine. In addition, it is possible for prescribers to prescribe diazepam on instalment prescriptions for the management of side effects to addiction treatment.

As it may not be desirable to supply patients addicted to drugs with a large quantity of a drug substitute, it is possible to supply the drug in instalments via specific instalment prescription forms. These prescription forms are similar to standard NHS prescription forms; however, they contain an extra portion for the pharmacist or pharmacy technician to record the details of each instalment.

Any pattern of instalments on an instalment prescription is permitted, although (for England and Wales) prescribers should limit their supply to 14 days (30 days for Scotland). For details of the different drugs that may be prescribed in instalments for England, Scotland and Wales, see *Medicines, Ethics and Practice: A guide for pharmacists and pharmacy technicians*.

A specific start date may be specified; if it is specified it must be followed. If no start date is specified, then a prescription may legally be started any time within the 28 days, but professionally we would be concerned if there was a gap in treatment.

Until recently there was a strict rule that instalments could be collected only on the day specified. However, if the prescriber includes the following wording (or similar wording approved by the Home Office) on the prescription then exceptions can be made:

Instalment prescriptions covering more than one day should be collected on the specified day; if this collection is missed the remainder of the instalment (i.e. the instalment less the amount prescribed for the day(s) missed) may be supplied.

Requisitions for controlled drugs

Requisitions for controlled drugs follow the same basic format as for other written requisitions. The following individuals may be supplied with a Schedule 2 or 3 controlled drug via a written requisition:

- a practitioner (doctor, dentist or vet)
- the matron or acting matron of a hospital or nursing home: the requisition must be signed by a doctor or dentist employed there
- a sister or acting sister in charge of a ward, theatre, or other hospital or nursing home
- a person in charge of a laboratory used for scientific education or research
- the owner or master of a British ship: where there is no doctor employed on board
- the installation manager of an offshore installation
- the master of a foreign ship in a port in the UK (note extra requirements apply)
- a supplementary prescriber.

KeyPoints

The following requirements apply to requisitions for Schedule 2 or 3 controlled drugs:
- Must be signed by the recipient (i.e. the person authorised to be supplied).
- State:
  - name
  - address
  - profession or occupation.
- Specify total quantity of drug and purpose for which it is required.
- The supplier must be satisfied that signature and qualification are genuine.

Requisitions for controlled drugs within the community

All requisitions for Schedules 2 and 3 controlled drugs, against which supplies are made by pharmacists from a community pharmacy, are now sent to the PPD (or equivalent) at the end of the month (in a similar way to NHS prescriptions). However, this is not for reimbursement (as the pharmacist or pharmacy technician will have charged the recipient to cover the cost of the medication and supply), but for monitoring purposes. In addition, the pharmacy should keep a photocopy of the requisition. This requirement does not currently apply to requisitions by veterinary practitioners or veterinary surgeons.

Once the requisition has been fulfilled, the pharmacist or pharmacy technician should mark the requisition with the name and address of the supplying pharmacy (e.g. stamp the requisition with the pharmacy stamp) and the date of supply.

The recording of the supply of Schedule 2 controlled drugs in the prescription-only medicines (POM) register against a written requisition is just a good practice requirement because an entry is made detailing the supply in the controlled drugs register. In addition, although you send the original requisition to the PPD (or equivalent) at the end of the month, you would still have a photocopy. For Schedule 3 controlled drugs, a POM register entry is also just good practice because you keep a photocopy of the original requisition form.

From 1 January 2008, standardised requisition forms were introduced in England (FP10CDF), Scotland (CDRF) and Wales (WP10CDF) for the ordering of Schedules 2 and 3 controlled drugs, and it is good practice for practitioners to use these forms when requisitioning Schedules 2 and 3 controlled drugs for human use from a community pharmacy. In exceptional circumstances, where a form other than the standardised requisition is used, there is still a legal requirement to submit the original requisition to the PPD (or equivalent) and to retain a copy.

Although it is not a legal requirement to provide a requisition where one community pharmacy supplies another community pharmacy, as good practice a written requisition should be obtained. This requisition should also be submitted to the PPD (or equivalent) for processing. A specific form for use by one community pharmacy to obtain stock from another community pharmacy has been developed in Scotland and should be used for this purpose.

A pharmacist may supply a controlled drug to a *practitioner* (and only a practitioner) in advance of requisition in an emergency. The pharmacist must receive the requisition within 24 hours of the supply. Messengers (e.g. a receptionist from the surgery) must have letter of authorisation in order to be in legal possession of the drugs.

Record keeping

Receipts and supplies of all Schedule 2 controlled drugs need to be recorded in the controlled drugs register. Currently, in most pharmacies, this is in the form of a bound book. Recent changes to the legislation have enabled the legal use of electronic controlled drugs registers, although suitable computer software is only just being developed. In the future, all controlled drugs registers will be electronic (as this facilitates audit of the use of controlled drugs).

KeyPoints

Receipts and supplies of all Schedule 2 controlled drugs need to be recorded in the controlled drugs register:

- Entries must be in ink or otherwise indelible.
- Entries must be in date order, i.e. chronological.
- Entries must be made on day of transaction or the following day.
- No cancellation, alteration or obliteration.
- The register entry must be made for each quantity supplied.
- The register must be kept at the premises at all times during use and for 2 years from the last date of entry.
- A separate register/part of the register is used for each class of drugs, and the class must be specified at the top of each page (although see below for additional requirements).
- Register, documents and stocks of drugs must be available for inspection.
- A record of whether the collector was the patient, the patient's representative or a healthcare professional (name and address need to be recorded) should be noted in the controlled drugs register.
- Pharmacists should make a record of whether or not they asked for proof of identity of individuals collecting Schedule 2 controlled drugs and whether proof of identity was provided.
- All controlled drugs registers should contain a running balance.

Storage

KeyPoints

The parts of the Misuse of Drugs regulations relating to the storage of controlled drugs within pharmacies are as follows:

- a cabinet built to specification in the regulations
- safe custody regulations apply to all Schedules 1 and 2 controlled drugs, except secobarbital (quinalbarbitone)
- safe custody regulations also apply to Schedule 3 controlled drugs but all drugs used are exempt, apart from buprenorphine, diethylpropion, flunitrazepam and temazepam.

Destruction

Controlled drugs to be destroyed need to be separated into those that are in the pharmacy stock and patient-returned controlled drugs. Different regulations apply to each situation and further details can be found in *Applied Pharmaceutical Practice* (Langley and Belcher, 2008) and *Medicines, Ethics and Practice: A guide for pharmacists and pharmacy technicians*.

Worked examples

Example 6.1

You receive prescription shown in Figure 6.1 in your pharmacy.

Figure 6.1

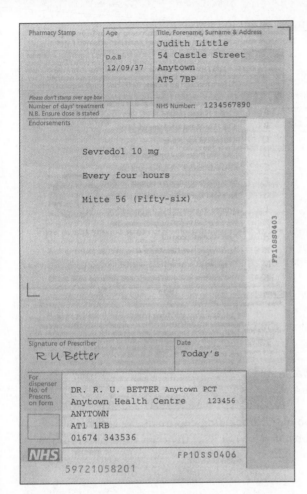

FP10SS0403

Inside the prescription form:

Pharmacy Stamp | Age | Title, Forename, Surname & Address

D.o.B
12/09/37

Judith Little
54 Castle Street
Anytown
AT5 7BP

Please don't stamp over age box
Number of days' treatment
N.B. Ensure dose is stated

NHS Number: 1234567890

Endorsements

Sevredol 10 mg

Every four hours

Mitte 56 (Fifty-six)

Signature of Prescriber | Date
R U Better | Today's

For dispenser No. of Prescns. on form

DR. R. U. BETTER Anytown PCT
Anytown Health Centre   123456
ANYTOWN
AT1 1RB
01674 343536

NHS   FP10SS0406
59721058201

1. Identity of order
NHS prescription (FP10SS). The prescription is for a drug that is classified as a Schedule 2 controlled drug. Therefore, the additional requirements relating to Schedule 2 controlled drugs need to be met before the prescription can be dispensed.

2. Prescriber
Doctor (general practitioner).

3. Legally written?
No. As the prescription is for a Schedule 2 controlled drug, additional prescription requirements need to be met before the prescription can be dispensed. In this case, the form of the prescription item and the full dosage instructions are missing (note that 'every 4 hours' is not sufficient, whereas 'one every 4 hours' would be).

Return the prescription to the prescriber for the form of the preparation and the full dosage instructions to be added.

4. Clinical check (complete Table 6.1)

Table 6.1

Drug	Indications	Dose check	Reference
Morphine (Sevredol)	Chronic pain	5–20 mg every 4 h adjusted according to response	*British National Formulary,* 56th edn, section 4.7.2

5. Interactions
There is only one drug on the prescription. However, it would also be advisable for the pharmacist or pharmacy technician to check the patient's medication record (PMR) for any concurrent medication that could cause an interaction.

6. Suitability for patient
The item prescribed is safe and suitable for an adult patient and the dose ordered on the prescription is within the recommended dose limits.

7. Item(s) allowable on the NHS
Yes (see *Drug Tariff*).

8. Records to be made (including copies of the record[s])
An entry would need to be made in the relevant section of the controlled drugs register detailing the supply. In addition a note of the intervention on a clinical intervention form would be made (Figure 6.2).

Figure 6.2

DRUG CLASS Morphine

NAME (brand, strength, form) Sevredol 10 mg tablets

Date supply received or date supplied	Obtained			Supplied							Balance
	Name, address of person or firm from whom obtained	Amount Obtained		Name, address of person or firm supplied	Authority to possess- prescriber or licence holder details	Person collecting Patient/Representative or Healthcare Professional (name and address)	Proof of identity requested Yes/No	Proof of identity provided Yes/No	Amount supplied		Carried over: 112
Today's				Judith Little 54 Castle Street Anytown	Dr R U Better FP10	Patient	Yes	Yes	56		56

9. Process prescription (including example of label[s])

- Prepare label for product.
- Check appendix 9 of *British National Formulary* for supplementary labelling requirements:
  - Sevredol: *British National Formulary* label number 2 (Warning: may cause drowsiness. If affected do not drive or operate machinery. Avoid alcoholic drink.)
- Select pack of Sevredol from the controlled drugs cupboard, remembering to check the expiry date and taking care that the correct strength of drug has been selected (the packaging of other strengths is very similar).
- Perform final check of item, label and prescription.
- Pack in a suitable bag ready to give to the patient or patient's representative (as this is a Schedule 2 controlled drug, it should be kept in the controlled drugs cupboard until it is collected by the patient or her representative).

Labels (we have assumed that the name and address of the pharmacy and the words 'Keep out of the reach and sight of children' are pre-printed on the label) (Figure 6.3).

Figure 6.3

Sevredol 10 mg Tablets	56
Take ONE tablet every four hours when required.	
Warning. May cause drowsiness.	
If affected do not drive or operate machinery.	
Avoid alcoholic drink.	
Ms Judith Little	Date of dispensing

10. Endorse prescription

Stamp with pharmacy stamp to indicate completion and mark the date of supply.

11. Destination of paperwork

Send to the PPD at the end of the month. The controlled drugs register in which the details of the supply were made must be kept at the premises at all times during use and for 2 years from the last date of entry.

12. Identity check/counselling

- Check patient's name and address.
- The pharmacist or pharmacy technician must identify whether the collector is the patient, patient's representative or a healthcare professional. This information (including the name and professional address if the collector is a healthcare professional) must be recorded in the controlled drugs register.
- The pharmacist or pharmacy technician must note, in the controlled drugs register, whether ID was requested from the collector and whether it was produced.

- The collector should be asked to sign the rear of the prescription form.
- Reinforce the dosage instructions; advise that the tablets are best taken every 4 hours as required and may cause drowsiness.
- Draw patient's attention to the patient information leaflet (PIL) and ask if she has any questions.

Example 6.2

You receive prescription shown in Figure 6.4 in your pharmacy.

Figure 6.4

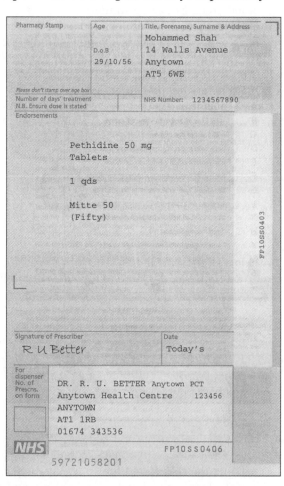

Pharmacy Stamp	Age	Title, Forename, Surname & Address
	D.o.B 29/10/56	Mohammed Shah 14 Walls Avenue Anytown AT5 6WE

Please don't stamp over age box

Number of days' treatment
N.B. Ensure dose is stated

NHS Number: 1234567890

Endorsements

Pethidine 50 mg
Tablets

1 qds

Mitte 50
(Fifty)

FP10SS0403

Signature of Prescriber

R U Better

Date

Today's

For dispenser No. of Prescns. on form

DR. R. U. BETTER Anytown PCT
Anytown Health Centre   123456
ANYTOWN
AT1 1RB
01674 343536

NHS

FP10SS0406

59721058201

1. Identity of order

NHS prescription (FP10SS). The prescription is for a drug that is classified as a Schedule 2 controlled drug. Therefore, the additional requirements relating to Schedule 2 controlled drugs need to be met before the prescription can be dispensed.

2. Prescriber
Doctor (general practitioner).

3. Legally written?
Yes. As the prescription is for a Schedule 2 controlled drug, additional prescription requirements need to be met before the prescription can be dispensed. In this case, all the additional legal requirements for a prescription for a Schedule 2 controlled drug have been met.

4. Clinical check (complete Table 6.2)

Table 6.2

Drug	Indications	Dose check	Reference
Pethidine	Acute pain	50–150 mg every 4 h	British National Formulary, 56th edn, section 4.7.2

5. Interactions
There is only one drug on the prescription. However, it would also be advisable for the pharmacist or pharmacy technician to check the PMR for any concurrent medication that could cause an interaction.

6. Suitability for patient
The item prescribed is safe and suitable for an adult patient and the dose ordered on the prescription is within the recommended dose limits.

7. Item(s) allowable on the NHS
Yes (see *Drug Tariff*).

8. Records to be made (including copies of the record[s])
An entry would need to be made in the relevant section of the controlled drugs register detailing the supply.

In this case, on checking your stock, it is noted that you only have 20 tablets available. Therefore, you would need to supply 20 now and inform the patient or the patient's representative that you will order the remainder of the prescription for collection when it arrives. The supply of the remaining 30 tablets would need to be made within the 28-day validity period of the prescription.

You will need to make an entry in the controlled drugs register for each supply made and mark the date of each supply on the prescription (Figure 6.5).

Figure 6.5

MISUSE OF DRUGS ACT
REGISTER OF:

DRUG CLASS   Pethidine

NAME (brand, strength, form)   Pethidine 50 mg tablets

Date	Obtained		Supplied							Balance
supply received or date supplied	Name, address of person or firm from whom obtained	Amount Obtained	Name, address of person or firm supplied	Authority to possess- prescriber or licence holder details	Person collecting Patient/Representative or Healthcare Professional (name and address)	Proof of identity requested Yes/No	Proof of identity provided Yes/No	Amount supplied		Carried over: 20
Today's			Mohammed Shah 14 Walls Avenue Anytown	Dr R U Better FP10	Patient	Yes	Yes	20		0
Date stock arrives	A Wholesaler 2 Supply Road Anytown	100								100
Date of supply			Mohammed Shah 14 Walls Avenue Anytown	Dr R U Better FP10	Patient	No	No	30		70

9. Process prescription (including example of label[s])

- Prepare label for product.
- Check appendix 9 of *British National Formulary* for supplementary labelling requirements:
  - Pethidine: *British National Formulary* label number 2 (Warning: may cause drowsiness. If affected do not drive or operate machinery. Avoid alcoholic drink.)
- Select pack of pethidine from the controlled drugs cupboard, remembering to check the expiry date.
- Perform final check of item, label and prescription.
- Pack in a suitable bag ready to give to the patient or his representative (as this is a Schedule 2 controlled drug, it should be kept in the controlled drugs cupboard until it is collected by the patient or his representative).

Labels (we have assumed that the name and address of the pharmacy and the words 'Keep out of the reach and sight of children' are pre-printed on the label) (Figure 6.6).

Figure 6.6

Pethidine 50 mg Tablets	20
Take ONE tablet FOUR times a day. Warning. May cause drowsiness. If affected do not drive or operate machinery. Avoid alcoholic drink.	
Mr Mohammed Shah	Date of dispensing

10. Endorse prescription

The date of the original supply (i.e. 20) needs to be marked on the prescription. If the patient or representative collects the remainder of the prescription (remember, they may not), then the date of this subsequent supply also needs to be marked on the prescription. In addition, before submission to the PPD (see below), the prescription needs to be stamped with the pharmacy stamp to indicate completion.

11. Destination of paperwork
Send to the PPD at the end of the month. The controlled drugs register in which the details of the supply were made must be kept at the premises at all times during use and for 2 years from the last date of entry.

12. Identity check/counselling
- Check patient's name and address.
- The pharmacist or pharmacy technician must identify whether the collector is the patient, patient's representative or a healthcare professional. This information (including the name and professional address if the collector is a healthcare professional) must be recorded in the controlled drugs register.
- The pharmacist or pharmacy technician must note in the controlled drugs register whether ID was requested from the collector and whether it was produced.
- The collector should be asked to sign the rear of the prescription form.
- Reinforce the dosage instructions; advise that the tablets may cause drowsiness.
- Inform the patient's representative that we owe some of the medication.
- Draw patient's representative's attention to the PIL and ask if he has any questions.

Self-assessment

Question 1
Drugs in which **ONE** of the following Schedules of the Misuse of Drugs Regulations would not routinely be prescribed in medical practice?
A Schedule 1
B Schedule 2
C Schedule 3
D Schedule 4
E Schedule 5

Question 2
Which **ONE** of the following is **NOT** a requirement on a requisition for a Schedule 2 controlled drug?
A Be signed by the recipient
B State the name of the recipient
C State the address of the recipient

QUANTITY?

D Specify the total quality of drug in both words and figures

E State the purpose for which the controlled drug has been requested

Question 3

Consider the following two statements:

1. The supply of a Schedule 3 controlled drug on a requisition does not need to be legally recorded in the POM register

because

2. A record of the supply would be made in a controlled drugs register.

Now indicate the **ONE CORRECT** alternative from options A–E below.

A Both statements are correct and statement 2 is the reason for statement 1

B Both statements are correct but statement 2 is not the reason for statement 1

C Statement 1 is correct but statement 2 is incorrect

D Statement 1 is incorrect but statement 2 is correct

E Neither statement 1 nor statement 2 is correct

Question 4

Which **ONE** of the following statements about instalment dispensing to drug addicts is **INCORRECT**?

A Any pattern of instalments is acceptable, but the pattern must be clearly stated on the prescription.

B A specific start date must be stated.

C Diamorphine, cocaine and dipipanone are disallowed as substitutes unless the doctor has a licence from the Home Office.

D Diazepam may also be prescribed on instalment prescriptions for treatment of drug addicts.

E Dextromoramide, morphine and pethidine are allowed as substitutes.

Questions 5–7 contain examples of prescription forms containing controlled drugs. The same standard systematic approach is followed as for other prescription forms. This approach is summarised in Chapter 3.

As before, complete the following sections to guide you through the dispensing process:

1. identity of order
2. prescriber
3. legally written?
4. clinical check (complete Table 6.3)
5. interactions
6. suitability for patient

7. item(s) allowable on the NHS
8. records to be made (including copies of the record(s))
9. process prescription (including example of label(s))
10. endorse prescription
11. destination of paperwork
12. identity check/counselling.

Table 6.3

Drug	Indications	Dose check	Reference

Question 5

You receive the prescription shown in Figure 6.7 in your pharmacy.

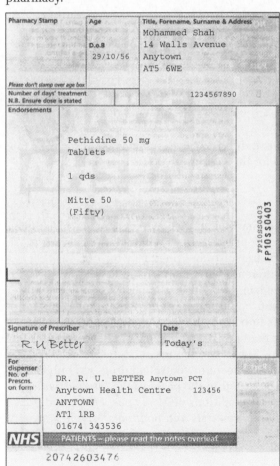

Figure 6.7

Using the sections indicated above, summarise all stages of the dispensing process for this prescription form.

Question 6
You receive the prescription shown in Figure 6.8 in your pharmacy.

Using the sections indicated above, summarise all stages of the dispensing process for this prescription form.

Figure 6.8

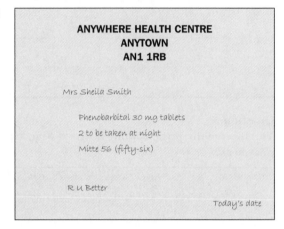

ANYWHERE HEALTH CENTRE
ANYTOWN
AN1 1RB

Mrs Sheila Smith

Phenobarbital 30 mg tablets
2 to be taken at night
Mitte 56 (fifty-six)

R U Better

Today's date

Question 7
You receive the prescription shown in Figure 6.9 in your pharmacy.

Using the sections indicated above, summarise all stages of the dispensing process for this prescription form.

Summary

This chapter has summarised all the key parts of the legislation relating to the use of controlled drugs within a pharmacy. It is important that all pharmacists and pharmacy technicians become familiar with the different requirements relating to how controlled drugs are handled within pharmacy as any deviation from the requirements could result in prosecution.

In addition, it is important that pharmacists and pharmacy technicians are aware of any developments or changes to the regulations that may be made in the future. Details of any updates or changes in the management of controlled drugs are published on the RPSGB's website and in the pages of the *Pharmaceutical Journal*. In addition, new editions of *Medicines, Ethics and Practice: A guide for pharmacists and pharmacy technicians* will

Figure 6.9

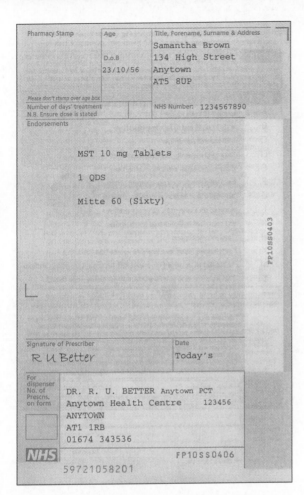

```
Pharmacy Stamp        Age          Title, Forename, Surname & Address
                                   Samantha Brown
                      D.o.B        134 High Street
                      23/10/56     Anytown
                                   AT5 8UP
Please don't stamp over age box
Number of days' treatment          NHS Number:  1234567890
N.B. Ensure dose is stated
Endorsements


         MST 10 mg Tablets

         1 QDS

         Mitte 60 (Sixty)

                                                    FP10SS0403




Signature of Prescriber            Date
R U Better                         Today's

For
dispenser
No. of      DR. R. U. BETTER Anytown PCT
Prescns.
on form     Anytown Health Centre     123456
            ANYTOWN
            AT1 1RB
            01674 343536
NHS                                FP10SS0406
         59721058201
```

collate all the recent changes. Pharmacies are expected to have standard operating procedures (SOPs) in place for all aspects of the management of controlled drugs and it is important that any changes in the regulations are also reflected in any SOPs in place.

chapter 7
Emergency supply

Overview

Upon completion of this chapter, you should be able to:

- understand the role of the pharmacist in the emergency supply of medication to both practitioners and patients
- make a legal emergency supply of a medicinal product at the request of a practitioner
- make a legal emergency supply of a prescription-only medicine at the request of a patient
- understand the role of patient group directions in the urgent supply of medication to patients in Scotland.

Introduction and overview

In addition to the supply of medication to patients against both NHS prescription forms in the community (see Chapters 2 and 3) and in a hospital setting (see Chapter 4), and private prescription forms (see Chapter 5), it may be necessary for pharmacists to supply medicines to patients, in an emergency, without a prescription form being present.

There are two types of emergency supply. Although colloquially they are both termed 'emergency supply', they are essentially very different. The two different forms of emergency supply are emergency supply at the request of a practitioner and emergency supply at the request of a patient. In addition, Scotland has implemented a system whereby patient group direction can be used in the urgent supply of medication to patients.

Emergency supply at the request of a practitioner

Essentially, this form of emergency supply is supply of medication in advance of a prescription form being supplied. It is the responsibility of the practitioner requesting the emergency supply to furnish the supplying pharmacist with a prescription form within 72 hours.

The following is the procedure for making an emergency supply at the request of a practitioner:

KeyPoints

Currently, emergency supplies at the request of a practitioner can be made only by one of the following UK-registered practitioners:

- doctors
- dentists
- community practitioner nurse prescribers
- supplementary prescribers
- nurse independent prescribers
- pharmacist independent prescribers.

- The pharmacist must be satisfied that the supply is being requested by a doctor, dentist, community practitioner nurse prescriber, supplementary prescriber, nurse independent prescriber or pharmacist independent prescriber.
- The pharmacist should remind the practitioner that it is his or her responsibility to furnish the prescription form within 72 hours.
- The item must not be a controlled drug in Schedule 1, 2 or 3 of the Misuse of Drugs Regulations (the only exception to this being phenobarbital or phenobarbital sodium for the treatment of epilepsy) (see Chapter 6).
- The item should be dispensed and labelled, as for any other supply, against a prescription form, according to the directions of the practitioner.
- An entry should be made in the prescription-only medicines (POM) register stating the following:
  - the date on which the emergency supply was made
  - the name, quantity and, except where it is apparent from the name, the pharmaceutical form and strength of the medicine; it is also good practice to record the dose and frequency of the medication
  - the name and address of the practitioner
  - the name and address of the patient.

When the prescription form is received, the pharmacist should add both the date on the prescription form and the date that the prescription form was received.

Therefore, all entries in the POM register relating to emergency supplies at the request of a practitioner will contain three dates:

1. The date that the emergency supply was made (i.e. supplied to the patient).
2. The date on the prescription form (once it has been received).
3. The date that the prescription form was received in the pharmacy.

All three dates should be present in the POM register, even if all three are the same.

It is also good practice, unless the medication is for a patient with whom you are familiar, to ask the practitioner for the age of the patient. This enables you to perform a suitable dose check. Remember that, just because the medication is being requested by a practitioner as an emergency supply, this does not negate the need for you to perform a suitable clinical check.

KeyPoints

The POM register entry for an emergency supply at the request of a practitioner must include the following pieces of information:

- the date on which the emergency supply was made
- the name, quantity and, except where it is apparent from the name, the pharmaceutical form and strength of the medicine; it is also good practice to record the dose and frequency of the medication
- the name and address of the practitioner
- the name and address of the patient.

When the prescription form is received, the pharmacist should add:

- the date on the prescription form
- the date that the prescription form was received.

Emergency supply at the request of a patient

Emergency supply at the request of a patient is very different from emergency supply at the request of a practitioner. In this case, as with the latter, there is no prescription form present at the time of supply of the POM. However, unlike emergency supply at the request of a practitioner, there is no prescription form to cover the supply provided at a later date. Remember that emergency supply of medication other than POMs (i.e. general sale list [GSL] or pharmacy-only [P] items) is not necessary because patients would be able to purchase these items from the pharmacy (so long as there was a clinical need).

The pharmacist making the emergency supply must have interviewed the patient making the request and be satisfied that:

- there is an immediate need for the POM and that the patient is unable to obtain a prescription form for the item within a reasonable time
- the item has been previously prescribed by a doctor, dentist, community practitioner nurse prescriber, supplementary prescriber, nurse independent prescriber or pharmacist independent prescriber
- the dose that the patient states would be appropriate for him or her to take
- the patient is taking no current medication with which the requested emergency supply would interact.

It is expected that the pharmacist would interview the patient in person in the pharmacy. However, in certain circumstances it may be impractical to do so and, on exceptional occasions, a telephone conversation, with any subsequent supply made via the patient's representative, may be appropriate.

If the pharmacist is satisfied that an emergency supply should be made, no more than 30 days' supply of the medication can be made, except in the following circumstances:

- Where it would be impractical to split a package (so long as the package has been made up in a container elsewhere than at the place of sale or supply), e.g. an emergency supply of an asthma inhaler.
- An oral contraceptive, where a full cycle may be supplied.
- An antibiotic in liquid form for oral administration where the smallest quantity to provide a full course of treatment may be supplied.

KeyPoints

The POM register entry for an emergency supply at the request of a patient should include the following pieces of information:

- the date on which the emergency supply was made
- the name, quantity and, except where it is apparent from the name, the pharmaceutical form and strength of the medicine; it is also good practice to include the dose and frequency of the medication and details of the patient's GP's name and address
- the name and address of the patient
- the nature of the emergency (i.e. why the patient requested the POM and why he or she could not obtain a prescription form).

- A controlled drug (i.e. phenobarbital or phenobarbital sodium for the treatment of epilepsy or any Schedule 4 or 5 controlled drug – see page 98) where a maximum of 5 days' treatment may be supplied.

Although the pharmacist can supply up to 30 days' treatment, consideration should be given to when the patient may be able realistically to obtain a prescription form and therefore it may be appropriate to supply less than 30 days' treatment.

The medication should be dispensed and labelled as normal, but in addition should include the words 'Emergency supply' on the label (often with the reference number of the POM register entry relating to the emergency supply).

As for emergency supplies at the request of a practitioner, emergency supplies at the request of a patient may not be for any controlled drugs in Schedules 1, 2 and 3 of the Misuse of Drugs Regulations (except phenobarbital or phenobarbital sodium for the treatment of epilepsy where supplies are limited to a maximum of 5 days' treatment) (see Chapter 6). In addition to these restrictions on emergency supplies, emergency supplies at the request of a patient may not be for medicines containing any of the following substances:

- ammonium bromide
- calcium bromide
- calcium bromidolactobionate
- embutramide
- fencamfamin hydrochloride
- fluanisone
- hexobarbital (hexobarbitone)
- hexobarbitone sodium
- hydrobromic acid
- meclofenoxate hydrochloride
- methohexital (methohexitone) sodium
- pemoline
- piracetam
- potassium bromide
- prolintane hydrochloride
- sodium bromide
- strychnine hydrochloride
- tacrine hydrochloride
- thiopental sodium.

The urgent supply of medicines or appliances to patients via patient group direction in Scotland

In Scotland an additional way of dealing with the urgent supply of medicines or appliances at the request of a patient to the emergency supply detailed above has been implemented using a patient group direction.

As with emergency supply of POMs in England and Wales, this patient group direction allows for the urgent supply of previously prescribed medicines that would normally be prescribed again once a supply had been exhausted. The urgent supply patient group direction was implemented in Scotland to allow patients to obtain supplies of routine medicines out of hours without having to contact out-of-hours services, especially over holiday periods.

For further details on the urgent supply of medicines or appliances to patients via patient group direction in Scotland, see *Applied Pharmaceutical Practice* (Langley and Belcher, 2008).

Worked examples

Example 7.1

It is Friday afternoon at around 4.00 pm. You receive a call in your pharmacy from a local doctor, Dr Ahmed, with whom you are familiar. He informs you that he is just visiting a patient under his care who requires some analgesics. Unfortunately, he has forgotten his prescription form pad and so is unable to write a prescription form for the supply. He is not returning to his surgery until Monday morning and so requests that you make an emergency supply of the analgesics. He will write a prescription form for the supply of the analgesics on Monday morning and place the prescription form in the post to you on Monday evening.

Should you make the emergency supply? The request is from a practitioner (Dr Ahmed) with whom you are familiar, so it is a reasonable request for you to supply the medication in this situation. You will need to know the following:

- the name and address (and if appropriate, the age) of the patient
- the name and address of the practitioner (although as you are familiar with Dr Ahmed you should have these details)
- details of the medication that the practitioner wishes the patient to take, including the name, form, strength, dose and frequency of the medication.

An entry will need to be made in the POM register stating the following:

- the date on which the emergency supply was made
- the name, quantity and, except where it is apparent from the name, the pharmaceutical form and strength of the medicine; it is also good practice to record the dose and frequency of the medication
- the name and address of the practitioner
- the name and address of the patient
- a space for (1) the date on the prescription form and (2) the date that the prescription form was received in the pharmacy.

In addition, it should be pointed out to Dr Ahmed that, if the prescription form is not posted to the pharmacy until Monday evening, even using first-class post, it may not arrive until Wednesday (if it is posted Monday evening, the post may not be collected until the following morning). This is longer than the 72 hours allowed for the prescriber to furnish you with a prescription form for the emergency supply. Although it is the prescriber's responsibility to ensure that you have the prescription form within 72 hours, it would be advisable for you to remind the prescriber of his or her responsibility at this point.

The POM register entry for this supply would appear in the register as shown in Figure 7.1. The label for this supply would look as shown in Figure 7.2 (we have assumed that the name and address of the pharmacy and the words 'Keep out of the reach and sight of children' are pre-printed on the label).

Figure 7.1

Reference number	Details		Cost
7.01 Date of supply	Emergency supply at the request of Dr Ahmed		Prescription charge (NHS or private) or details of exemption (NHS)
	Timothy Small	Dr Ahmed	
	137 Holly Avenue	The Health Centre	
	Anytown	Anytown	
	50 Co-codamol 30/500 tablets		
	2 QDS PRN		
	Date on prescription:		
	Date prescription form received:		

Figure 7.2

Co-codamol 30/500 Tablets	50

Take TWO tablets FOUR times a day when required.
Warning. May cause drowsiness.
If affected do not drive or operate machinery.
Avoid alcoholic drink.
Do not take more than 2 at any one time.
Do not take more than 8 in 24 hours.
Do not take with any other paracetamol products.

Mr Timothy Small	Date of dispensing

Example 7.2

It is Saturday afternoon at around 4.00 pm. A patient with whom you are familiar (Emma Fox) comes into the pharmacy and asks for your assistance. She suffers from asthma and has run out of her medication. Her doctor's surgery is closed at the weekend and the patient cannot obtain a prescription form until Monday morning. Should you make the emergency supply?

The request is from a patient with whom you are familiar. She is a regular patient of your pharmacy and upon examining her PMR you notice regular supplies of salbutamol. You will also be aware of the opening times of the local surgery and able to confirm that the surgery is closed until Monday morning. Therefore, it is a reasonable request for you to supply the medication in this situation. You need to interview the patient and ascertain the following:

- There is an immediate need for the POM and the patient is unable to obtain a prescription form for the item.
- The item has been previously prescribed by a doctor, dentist, community practitioner nurse prescriber, supplementary prescriber, nurse independent prescriber or pharmacist independent prescriber.
- The dose and frequency that the patient says she uses would be appropriate for her to take.
- Whether the patient is taking any other medication, to enable you to check that the requested emergency supply doesn't interact with any other medication currently being taken.

The patient states that she inhales two puffs of the salbutamol inhaler when required, usually not more than once a day. As this medicine is an inhaler, it is not possible to limit the supply to 30 days' treatment (it is not possible to split an inhaler into smaller units). Therefore, one inhaler must be supplied.

An entry needs to be made in the POM register stating the following:

- the date on which the emergency supply was made
- the name, quantity and, except where it is apparent from the name, the pharmaceutical form and strength of the medicine; it is also good practice to include the dose and frequency of the medication and details of the patient's GP's name and address
- the name and address of the patient
- the nature of the emergency (i.e. why the patient requested the POM and why she could not obtain a prescription form).

The POM register entry for this supply would appear in the register as shown in Figure 7.3. The label for this supply would look as shown in Figure 7.4 (we have assumed that the name and address of the pharmacy and the words 'Keep out of the reach and sight of children' are pre-printed on the label):

Figure 7.3

Reference number	Details		Cost
7.02 Date of supply	Emergency supply at the request of a patient		Cost of drug + % Mark-up + Professional Fee + VAT
	Emma Fox	Dr Ahmed	
	2 Midtown Rise	The Health Centre	
	Anytown	Anytown	
	1 salbutamol inhaler		
	2 puffs to be inhaled when required		
	The patient suffers from asthma and has run out of medication. The request was made on Saturday afternoon and it is impractical for the patient to obtain a prescription form before Monday morning.		

Figure 7.4

> **Salbutamol 100 mcg Inhaler**   1
>   Inhale TWO puffs when required.
>   Emergency Supply (7.02).
> Mrs Emma Fox   Date of dispensing

Self-assessment

Question 1
A doctor requests an emergency supply for a patient. Which **ONE** of the following is legally required to be recorded in the POM register?
A   Age of the patient
B   Dose of the medication
C   Date on which the prescription is received
D   The words 'Emergency supply at the request of a doctor'
E   The doctor's qualifications

Question 2
Which **ONE** of the following medications could **NOT** legally be supplied to a patient at his or her request in an emergency?
A   Diazepam 5 mg tablets
B   Buprenorphine 200 microgram tablets
C   Codeine phosphate 15 mg tablets
D   Erythromycin suspension 250 mg/5 mL
E   Beclometasone 200 micrograms MDI

Question 3

When a POM is supplied to a patient following an emergency supply at the request of a doctor, which ONE of the following does NOT need to be printed on the label?

A   The name and strength of the medication
B   The name of the patient
C   The directions for use
D   The date of supply
E   The words 'Emergency supply'

Question 4

Which ONE of the following practitioners is NOT legally entitled to request an emergency supply for a patient?

A   Veterinary surgeon
B   Independent nurse prescriber
C   Community practitioner nurse prescriber
D   Pharmacist independent prescriber
E   Pharmacist supplementary prescriber

Each of questions 5–7 consists of two statements. You need to:

- decide whether the first statement is true or false
- decide whether the second statement is true or false
- then choose:

A   If both statements are true and the second statement is a correct explanation of the first statement.
B   If both statements are true but the second statement is NOT a correct explanation of the first statement.
C   If the first statement is true but the second statement is false.
D   If the first statement is false but the second statement is true.
E   If both statements are false.

Question 5

Mr John Smith, a regular patient, asks you if you could supply him with phenobarbital 60 mg tablets that he needs to control his epilepsy. He explains that he has accidentally run out of tablets and as it is Saturday morning the earliest he could see his doctor for a prescription is Monday morning.
Statement 1: You cannot lawfully issue the emergency supply.
Statement 2: Phenobarbital is a Schedule 3 controlled drug.

Question 6

Mr Drillett, the local dentist, telephones to ask you to provide an emergency supply of four tinidazole tablets 500 mg for Miss Sally Tooth because she needs treatment for an acute attack of ulcerative gingivitis. He is unable to provide a prescription immediately as he is dealing with another patient but his nurse will bring a prescription to you later in the afternoon.

Statement 1: You cannot lawfully issue the emergency supply for Miss Tooth.

Statement 2: Tinidazole tablets are not included in the *Dental Practitioner's Formulary*.

Question 7

Mr Downes visits your pharmacy and asks if you could let him have a salbutamol inhaler for his wife Connie because she lost her inhaler while shopping and the doctor's surgery is closed until Monday morning. He is concerned because she needs to use it once or twice every day. Connie is a regular patient and the PMR confirms that the item has been ordered before at the dose suggested and you feel that there is an immediate need for the medication.

Statement 1: You cannot legally issue the emergency supply for Mrs Downes.

Statement 2: Mr Downes is not the patient.

For questions 8–10, **ONE** or **MORE** of the responses/statements is/are correct regarding emergency supplies. Decide which of the responses/statements is/are correct and then choose:

A   If statements 1, 2 and 3 are all correct
B   If statements 1 and 2 are correct and statement 3 is incorrect
C   If statements 2 and 3 are correct and statement 1 is incorrect
D   If statement 1 is correct and statements 2 and 3 are incorrect
E   If statement 3 is correct and statements 1 and 2 are incorrect

Question 8

1. All medicines supplied as an emergency should be labelled 'Emergency supply'.
2. It is illegal for a community pharmacy to make an emergency supply to a patient without first contacting the patient's GP.
3. In general no more than 30 days' treatment may be sold or supplied for an emergency supply at the request of a patient.

Question 9

1. It is illegal to supply Schedule 1 or 2 controlled drugs as an emergency supply.
2. The pharmacist must make an entry in the POM register every time that an emergency supply is made.
3. If 30 days' supply of the medication is insufficient (following an emergency supply at the request of a patient), the patient may be advised to obtain a further supply from a different pharmacy.

Question 10
1. When making an emergency supply the pharmacist must be satisfied that it is a genuine emergency.
2. The emergency supply regulations permit the pharmacist to give only 5 days' supply of an oral contraceptive for an emergency supply at the request of a patient.
3. If an emergency supply at the request of a patient is made against the promise of an NHS prescription, this must be supplied within 72 hours.

Summary

In summary, the following key points relate to emergency supply.
1. There are two distinctly different types of emergency supply:
   (a) emergency supply at the request of a practitioner (in effect, supply of medication in advance of a prescription form)
   (b) emergency supply (of POM) at the request of a patient (where no prescription form will be provided)
   (c) although both are termed 'emergency supply', they are essentially very different and it is important that pharmacists and pharmacy technicians become familiar with both types.
2. In both cases, an entry in the POM register is made. This provides details of, and reason for, the supply.
3. The emergency supply of Schedule 1, 2 or 3 controlled dugs is prohibited except phenobarbital and phenobarbital sodium for the treatment of epilepsy.
4. For emergency supply at the request of a patient, up to 30 days' supply may be made (except in certain circumstances) (see also point 5). However, consideration should be given to supplying enough for fewer than 30 days. Emergency supply at the request of a practitioner has no supply limit, although professional judgement should be exercised if the requested quantity appears excessive.
5. In addition to the traditional emergency supply, additional arrangements exist within Scotland to allow the urgent supply of medicines or appliances to patients via patient group direction.

Overview

Upon completion of this chapter, you should be able to:

- revise the key points behind effective interpersonal communication
- learn how to undertake successful verbal communication
- appreciate the importance of non-verbal communication
- realise the role of body language in both verbal and non-verbal communication
- understand the different types of questioning that can be used
- be aware of the role that questioning mnemonics can play in effective patient communication
- learn how important listening and clear explanation can be.

Introduction and overview

The supply of medication to a patient is an important role for pharmacy. However, in addition to the actual supply, sufficient information needs to be given to the patient or the patient's carer to enable that patient to use the medicine safely and effectively. Although it is important to supply the correct medication to the patient, unless it is used correctly by the patient it may be ineffectual. In extreme cases, this can lead to patient harm or even death.

In addition to information being supplied to the patient in a printed format (i.e. via the medicine's label and the patient information leaflet [PIL]), it is often the role of the pharmacist or pharmacy technician to verbally counsel the patient or the patient's carer and demonstrate the use of the medication. Therefore, it is vital that

KeyPoints

Sending a message – in order to ensure that a message is received correctly, the message *sender* needs to:

- speak clearly
- speak slowly
- use appropriate language
- check understanding.

Receiving a message – in order to ensure that a message is received correctly, the message *receiver* needs to:

- listen carefully
- ask for clarification
- write it down
- repeat the message back in order to check that the message received is the one given.

A message consists of:

- *factual* information transmitted *verbally*
- *feeling* or *emotional* information transmitted *non-verbally*.

pharmacists and pharmacy technicians develop effective communication skills.

This chapter reinforces the basics of patient communication. Chapter 9 recaps specific details of the important counselling points that need to be considered for specific dosage forms. Further in-depth discussion of the material found in these two chapters can be found in *Applied Pharmaceutical Practice* (Langley and Belcher, 2008).

Verbal communication is purely the linguistic element of the message and includes the following:

- **Vocabulary**: using appropriate vocabulary and avoiding the use of jargon. Often words that are second nature to you may be totally alien to the patient. An example of this would be if a pharmacist or pharmacy technician advised a patient that a 'PIL' is enclosed with their medication, instead of saying that a 'patient information leaflet' is enclosed. To patients the term 'PIL' is more likely to mean a pharmaceutical form (a pill) and, although incorrectly interpreted, they will probably think of a tablet or more probably the contraceptive pill.
- **Use of language**: be aware of, and avoid, what has been referred to as 'restricted language code', which makes use of colloquial expressions, shorter and simpler sentences, repetitive use of conjunctions (but, because, so . . .) and the use of statements phrased as questions: 'Know what I mean?', '. . . you know?', '. . . isn't it?', etc. However, occasionally you may need to apply restricted language code when interacting with certain patients to ensure that the information is clearly understood.

KeyPoints

There are five main areas of body language:
(1) gaze or eye contact
(2) facial expression
(3) proximity and orientation
(4) posture
(5) touch.

Non-verbal communication could be defined as all forms of human communication except for the purely verbal message, i.e. the words themselves.

Vocal non-verbal communication includes the tone, pitch, volume, accent, speed, etc. and this is known as paralanguage. The meaning of a phrase can alter with the changing emphasis placed on the words in the phrase.

Questioning

There are six types of questions:
(1) closed questions
(2) open questions
(3) leading/biased questions
(4) probing questions
(5) prompting questions
(6) multiple questions.
It is important to use the right type of question to elicit the information required.

Questioning mnemonics

The importance of questioning patients correctly cannot be underestimated. The information from the patient is vital when 'responding to symptoms', so the interaction needs to be structured in order to ensure that all the relevant details are obtained.

How do you ensure that your interview with a patient is unbiased and thorough? How do you make sure that you don't forget to ask something? Your decision with regard to counter prescribing or referral to a general practitioner is based on the information that you manage to obtain from the patient.

As a result of the importance of remembering all the information, a number of mnemonics are used. These are valuable as a starting point; all the information is valid and you can build upon the framework to obtain further information from a patient. However, no mnemonic is fully comprehensive.

WWHAM

Who is the medicine for?
What are the symptoms?
How long have you been ill?
Action taken so far?
Medicines being taken at the moment?

This system of questioning establishes the presenting complaint and also gives information about what the patient has already done about the symptoms. However, it fails to consider family history, previous symptoms, general appearance or any social or lifestyle factors associated with the presenting symptoms.

For example, if these were the only questions used to differentiate between patients, a young mum presenting with indigestion/heartburn caused by a hectic lifestyle with poor eating habits ('eating on the go') might be given the same treatment as an elderly man presenting with similar symptoms, but with a greater chance of the symptoms being caused by a disease state rather than poor eating habits.

ENCORE

> Explore
> No medication?
> Care
> Observe
> Refer
> Explain

- **Explore**: this gives the opportunity to obtain information about the nature of the symptoms, discover any other associated symptoms or any other medication being taken by the patient, and hence any other pre-existing medical conditions; as a result of our 'exploration' we may exclude the possibility of serious disease. It also enables the questioner to obtain the identity of the patient.
- **No medication**: this is a reminder that medication is not always the answer and lifestyle changes may be more advisable – there is not necessarily 'a pill for all ills'.
- **Care**: this is to remind us that different patients have different needs. The needs of some categories are greater, e.g. children and elderly patients may be special cases, as would pregnant and breast-feeding women. These factors may well influence the recommendations made by pharmacists or pharmacy technicians.
- **Observe**: this is particularly important when attempting diagnosis.
- **Refer**: this is to remind you that you can refer a patient for a second opinion. Usually referral is advised if the patients are at increased risk, e.g. children, elderly patients, or if the symptoms are persistent or suggest a potentially serious condition.
- **Explain**: this is to remind us to fully explain decisions to patients. If a course of action is clearly explained the patient is more likely to be compliant.

With this system of questioning you do take into account the appearance of the patient. Careful observation of a patient can reveal a lot. If a patient presenting with symptoms is seriously ill, he or she rarely looks well. If you define what you think are observable symptoms of ill health you could include flushing, sweating, dilated pupils or smell. 'N' (for no medication) and 'R' (for refer), although they are relevant, do not really help towards making differential diagnosis. Once again no social or lifestyle factors are considered, and neither is family history taken into account.

AS METTHOD

> Age of the patient?
> Self or someone else?
> Medicines the patient is taking?

Exactly what does the patient mean by the symptom?

Time/duration of the symptom?

Taken anything for it or seen the doctor?

History of any disease or condition?

Other symptoms being experienced?

Doing anything to aggravate or alleviate the condition?

This system establishes the presenting complaint and whether or not the patient has had it before. It can be used to find the necessary information for making a diagnosis. Remember that not all questions will necessarily need to be asked and that the order of questioning is not that critical. Use the mnemonic as a checklist or *aide memoire*.

SIT DOWN SIR

Site or location?

Intensity or severity?

Type or nature?

Duration?

Onset?

With? (Other symptoms)

N annoyed or aggravated by?

Spread or radiation?

Incidence or frequency pattern?

Relieved by?

This mnemonic may help to elicit more information, it establishes severity, nature of symptoms and previous history, but again the importance of social or lifestyle factors is ignored as is the general appearance of the patient.

Try using these mnemonics in the scenario above that demonstrated the use of different types of questions. Were all the points covered?

Although these mnemonics are a useful aid or memory jogger they are not a replacement for clinical consultation; they should aid your decision-making but not constrain it.

Listening

Listening involves both verbal and non-verbal communication. There are different levels of listening and, as explained earlier, what we say isn't always what is heard, so conversely do we always hear what a patient is saying to us?

- **'Half-an-ear listening'**: this is background noise listening; we can hear the radio in the background but are we really listening to it?
- **'Passive listening'**: also known as 'stunned mullet' listening (an Australian term), this refers to a listener who is showing a vacant expression or completely blank look, and gives the speaker no feedback. This is useful for calming people down

but hopefully is not the type of listening that occurs in a pharmacy.

- **'Reflective listening'**: here the listener reflects the statements back to the speaker to encourage him or her to carry on with the thread of conversation; this is the type of listening employed by psychiatrists and counsellors.
- **'Active listening'**: this is the main type of listening used in pharmacy in responding to symptom scenarios.

The listening process can be divided into six distinct sections:

1. Concentrating, organising and analysing what is said. This may seem obvious but the process can be hindered in a number of ways.
2. Processing any information that is provided by a patient and perhaps altering the pattern of the consultation to accommodate any newly arising issues. Words don't always paint a true picture: listen to the underlying message that is conveyed by 'feelings' or 'emotions'.
3. Approaching patients with an open mind.
4. Listening with eyes as well as ears.
5. Do not interrupt a patient; let him or her finish before you speak.
6. Acknowledging the patient by showing him or her that you are listening.

Remember, all the benefits of effective communication will be lost if the pharmacist then fails to explain the use of the recommended treatment.

Explanation

When responding to symptoms in the pharmacy it is important to clearly explain the decision taken to the patient. Perhaps even more crucial is explanation of the purpose and use of prescribed or over-the-counter medicines. Pharmacists and pharmacy technicians are the last link in the prescribing chain. We are responsible for ensuring that the correct medicine is dispensed and it is important that we make certain that the patient knows how to take it correctly. Part of the pharmacist's and pharmacy technician's role is to help patients overcome any confusion that they may have with respect to their medication.

KeyPoints

Remember, there are three parts to a good explanation:
1. planning
2. presentation
3. feedback.

Self-assessment

Question 1
Which **ONE** of the following statements is **NOT** part of the mnemonic ENCORE?

A   E stands for 'Explore'
B   C stands for 'Care'
C   O stands for 'Other symptoms'
D   R stands for 'Refer'

Question 2
Which **ONE** of the following statements is **NOT** part of the mnemonic AS METTHOD?

A   D stands for 'Doing anything to aggravate or alleviate the condition'
B   E stands for 'Exactly what does the patient mean by the symptom'
C   A stands for 'Age of the patient'
D   H stands for 'History of medicines taken'

Question 3
Which **ONE** of the following statements is **NOT** part of the mnemonic WWHAM?

A   W stands for 'Who is the medicine for?'
B   W stands for 'What medicines have been tried?'
C   H stands for 'How long have you been ill?'
D   M stands for 'Medicines being taken at the moment?'

Question 4
Which **ONE** of the following statements is **NOT** part of the mnemonic SIT DOWN SIR?

A   S stands for 'Site or location'
B   T stands for 'Type or nature'
C   D stands for 'Doing anything to alleviate the condition'
D   O stands for 'Onset'

Question 5
Which **ONE** of the following questions is a closed question?

A   What is your name?
B   What exactly are the symptoms?
C   What do you mean?
D   How often do you take the tablets?

Question 6

Which **ONE** of the following types of question gives a patient the opportunity to give full answers?

A   Closed questions
B   Open questions
C   Leading questions
D   Probing questions

Question 7

When listening to a patient which **ONE** of the following actions would be inappropriate?

A   Acknowledge the patient
B   Avoid eye contact
C   Concentrate on information provided by the patient
D   Allow the patient to finish before speaking

The following questions require the use of *Applied Pharmaceutical Practice* (Langley and Belcher, 2008) and other additional reference sources, in addition to this text.

Question 8

Which **ONE** of the following symptoms of headache does NOT suggest referral to a doctor?

A   Fever
B   Slurred speech
C   Neck stiffness
D   Drowsiness with visual disturbances and vomiting

Question 9

Which **ONE** of the following symptoms of cough does **NOT** suggest referral to a doctor?

A   Chest pain
B   Child with night-time cough not associated with a common cold
C   Blood in sputum
D   Non-productive, dry, tickly cough associated with a cold

Question 10

Which **ONE** of the following symptoms of vaginal candidiasis does **NOT** suggest referral to a doctor?

A   Vaginal discharge
B   Abdominal pain
C   Diabetes
D   Pregnancy

Question 11

Which **ONE** of the following laxatives would be the most appropriate for the treatment of an elderly bedridden man?

A   **Bisacodyl**
B   **Senna**
C   **Lactulose**
D   **Liquid paraffin**

For questions 12–20, **ONE** or **MORE** of the responses/statements is/are correct. Decide which of the responses/statements is/are correct and then choose:

A   If statements 1, 2 and 3 are all correct
B   If statements 1 and 2 are correct and statement 3 is incorrect
C   If statements 2 and 3 are correct and statement 1 is incorrect
D   If statement 1 is correct and statements 2 and 3 are incorrect
E   If statement 3 is correct and statements 1 and 2 are incorrect

Question 12

Diagnosis of head lice infestation is based on:

1.   **Detection of lice by combing**
2.   **Itchy scalp**
3.   **Cleanliness of hair**

Question 13

Which of the following statements about treatment of head lice infestation are true?

1.   **Alcoholic formulations are more effective.**
2.   **Alcoholic formulations should be avoided by people with asthma.**
3.   **Routine use of alcoholic formulations is recommended as prophylaxis.**

Question 14

Which of the following statements about cradle cap is/are true?

1.   **Cradle cap is a form of seborrhoeic dermatitis.**
2.   **Baby oil or olive oil could be used to relieve the condition.**
3.   **It is contagious.**

Question 15

Consider this scenario and decide which of the statements is/are correct. A patient in the pharmacy asks for treatment for hard skin on his foot. He thinks that it might be a corn; however, on examining the foot you find that it is a hard plaque of skin with a central black area situated on the sole of the foot.

1. Patient should be asked if he or she has diabetes.
2. A salicylic acid-containing treatment would be most appropriate.
3. No treatment should be offered and the patient should be referred immediately to his or her doctor.

Question 16

A mother asks your advice about chickenpox. Test your knowledge by stating which of these statements is/are correct?
1. Chickenpox is caused by herpes simplex virus.
2. Chickenpox can be contracted from contact with a patient with active shingles.
3. Promethazine is a drug that may alleviate some of the symptoms of chickenpox.

Question 17

Symptoms of tinea pedis include:
1. Itching
2. Mainly located between the toes
3. Skin appears white and macerated

Question 18

Concerning haemorrhoids, which of the following statements is/are correct?
1. Sitting on a hot radiator or a cold wall gives you piles.
2. Haemorrhoids (piles) are usually triggered by pregnancy or by straining as a result of childbirth or constipation.
3. If haemorrhoids have been present for more than 3 weeks this warrants referral.

Question 19

A pharmacist receives a prescription for Betnovate Cream, directions 'apply bd to hand'. The patient asks the pharmacist for further advice. The pharmacist should advise the patient to:
1. Apply sparingly (thinly)
2. Apply one fingertip unit
3. Cover the hand with a plastic glove after application

Question 20

A pharmacist receives a prescription for lactulose solution, directions '15 mL bd'. The patient asks the pharmacist for further advice. Which of the following statements would be suitable?
1. Some people find lactulose unpleasant to take so it may be mixed with water, fruit juice or squash.
2. May suffer from increased flatulence for the first few days.
3. Lactulose works in the same way as the Fybogel that you have had before.

Summary

This chapter has covered the basics of patient communication. It is important that pharmacists and pharmacy technicians are familiar with both verbal and non-verbal communication and able to communicate effectively with patients and carers.

chapter 9
Patient counselling and communication 2: product-specific counselling points

Overview

Upon completion of this chapter, you should be able to:
- understand the key counselling points relating to the following specific dosage forms:
  - ear drops and sprays
  - eye drops
  - eye ointments
  - inhalers
  - liquid oral dosage forms
  - nasal drops
  - nasal sprays
  - oral powders
  - patches
  - pessaries and vaginal creams
  - suppositories
  - tablets and capsules
  - topical applications.

Introduction and overview

Chapter 8 summarised the basics of patient communication, ensuring that pharmacists and pharmacy technicians are familiar with both verbal and non-verbal communication and able to communicate effectively with patients and carers. This chapter contains a recap on the key specific counselling points relating to the following dosage forms:
- ear drops and sprays
- eye drops
- eye ointments
- inhalers
- liquid oral dosage forms
- nasal drops
- nasal sprays

- oral powders
- patches
- pessaries and vaginal creams
- suppositories
- tablets and capsules
- topical applications.

Further details on each of the dosage forms contained within this chapter can be found in *Applied Pharmaceutical Practice* (Langley and Belcher, 2008) including the following:

- illustrations of some of the key dosage forms
- any special considerations, including illustrations of how the different dosage forms are used
- tips when using various different dosage forms
- special points for consideration with children
- details of different compliance aids.

Ear drops and sprays

1. Wash hands with soapy water before using the ear drops or spray.
2. Clean and dry the ear gently with a facecloth.
3. If necessary, shake the bottle of drops or spray. Some drops and sprays are suspensions and will need shaking; if applicable, this direction will be on the label.
4. Warm the ear drops or spray by holding the bottle in the hand for a few minutes.
5. Remove the lid.
6. Lie down on side with the affected ear uppermost (or tilt the head to one side).
7. Gently pull the ear lobe upwards and backwards, to straighten the ear canal.
8. Drop the drops or spray into the ear canal.
9. Gently massage just in front of the ear.
10. Stay lying down or with the head tilted for 5 minutes to allow the medication to run down the ear canal.
11. Return to the upright position and wipe away any excess medication.
12. Repeat if necessary in the other ear.
13. Replace the lid.

Eye drops

1. Wash hands with soapy water before using eye drops.
2. If necessary clean the eyes with boiled and cooled water and a tissue (one tissue for each eye) to remove any discharge or remaining wateriness (do not use cotton wool because it may leave fibres behind that could irritate the eye).

3. Shake the bottle of drops if necessary. Some eye drops are suspensions and will need shaking; if applicable, this direction will be on the label.
4. Remove the lid from the bottle.
5. Relax and either sit or lie down, tilting the head backwards so that you are looking at the ceiling.
6. Gently pull down the lower eyelid with a finger to make a pocket between the eye and the lower lid.
7. Look upwards.
8. Rest the dropper bottle on the forehead above the eye.
9. Squeeze one drop inside the lower eyelid (do not allow the dropper tip to touch the eye).
10. Close the eye and gently blot away any excess drops on a clean tissue.
11. Apply slight pressure to the inner corner of the eye for about 30 seconds. This prevents the drops running down the tear duct and into the back of the throat, avoiding any unpleasant aftertaste and also minimising any absorption into the body, so minimising possible side effects.
12. Replace the lid on the bottle.
13. Remember to discard any remaining drops 4 weeks after opening.

Eye ointments

1. Wash hands with soapy water before using eye ointment.
2. Clean your eye if necessary (as with eye drops – see above).
3. Sit in front of a mirror.
4. Remove the lid from the eye ointment.
5. Applying the ointment:
   - gently pull down the lower eyelid forming a pocket between the eyelid and the eye
   - hold the tube above the eye without touching it
   - gently squeeze the tube and place about 1 cm of ointment into the pocket, starting from nearest the nose to the outer edge
   - twist the wrist to break the strip of ointment from the tube
   - close the eye and blink to help spread the eye ointment over the eyeball; body temperature helps to melt the ointment so that it spreads over the surface of the eye
   - vision will be blurred for a few moments; keep blinking and the vision will clear
   - wipe away excess ointment using a clean tissue.
6. Replace the lid of the tube.
7. Remember to discard any remaining ointment 4 weeks after opening.

Inhalers

Inhalers are designed to help medication to be delivered directly into the lungs, where it will act mainly on the lung tissue and systemic effects will be minimised. The doses employed in inhalers are significantly less than the doses used in oral medication, so the incidence of side effects will also be reduced. There are a number of different types of inhaler available:

- metered dose inhalers (MDIs) – also called aerosol inhalers
- metered dose inhalers used with spacer attachment
- dry powder inhalers:
  - Turbohalers
  - Accuhalers
- breathe-actuated inhalers such as Easi-Breathe.

Metered dose inhalers

1. Remove the cap covering the mouthpiece and check that there is no fluff or dirt in the mouthpiece.
2. Shake the inhaler.
3. If the inhaler is new or has not been used for some time it will need to be tested. To test:
   - hold the inhaler away from body
   - press the top of the aerosol canister once
   - a fine mist should be puffed into the air
   - the inhaler is now ready to use.
4. Tilt head back slightly.
5. Breathe out gently.
6. Place the mouthpiece in the mouth between the teeth (do not bite). Close lips around the mouthpiece.
7. Start to breathe in slowly through the mouth; at the same time press down on the inhaler to release the medicine into the lungs.
8. Hold breath for between 5 and 10 seconds, then breathe out slowly.
9. If a second dose is required wait about 30 seconds and repeat the process.
10. Replace the cap and, if the inhaler is a corticosteroid inhaler, rinse the mouth out with water.

Metered dose inhalers used with spacer attachment

1. First assemble the spacer device if necessary as directed by the manufacturer (with or without a facemask).
2. Remove the cap from the inhaler and insert the mouthpiece of the inhaler into the opening at the end of the spacer.
3. Hold the spacer and inhaler together and shake.
4. Breathe out.

5. Put the spacer mouthpiece in the mouth and seal with the lips.
6. Press the inhaler once and then breathe in and out four or five times.
7. Further doses may be taken waiting a few seconds between puffs.
8. Separate the spacer and inhaler. Replace the inhaler cap and store until next dose.

Dry powder inhalers
Turbohalers
1. To load the Turbohaler before use:
   - unscrew the cover and remove it
   - hold the Turbohaler upright with one hand and with the other twist the grip in one direction as far as it will go
   - now twist back as far as it will go; a click should be heard showing that the inhaler is primed and ready for use.
2. Breathe out gently.
3. Place the mouthpiece between the lips and breathe in through the mouth as deeply and as hard as possible.
4. Remove the inhaler from the mouth and breathe out slowly.
5. Replace the lid.
6. Repeat the above steps if more than one puff is required.

Accuhalers
1. With the Accuhaler mouthpiece facing the patient, slide the lever away until it clicks. This will have loaded a dose ready for inhalation and the Accuhaler will move the dose counter on.
2. Hold the Accuhaler flat and breathe out away from the inhaler.
3. Seal lips around the Accuhaler mouthpiece and inhale deeply.
4. Remove inhaler form the mouth and hold breath as long as is comfortable.
5. Slide the thumb grip back towards patient to close the inhaler.
6. For further doses repeat above steps.

Easi-Breathe inhalers
1. Shake the inhaler.
2. Hold the inhaler upright and open the cap.
3. Breathe out, away from the inhaler.
4. Put the mouthpiece in the mouth and seal lips around it.
5. Breathe in steadily through the mouthpiece.
6. Hold breath for about 10 seconds.

7. Keeping the inhaler upright close the cap.
8. For further doses repeat the above steps.

Liquid oral dosage forms

The oral route of administration is the preferred route in the UK with tablets and capsules being the most common dosage forms. However, in certain cases liquids are required, particularly where a patient has swallowing difficulties or is a young child.

There are different types of liquid medicines including the following:

- **Solutions**: these include elixirs, syrups, linctuses and simple solutions, traditionally termed 'mixtures'.
- **Suspensions**: in this type of medicine insoluble solids are suspended in the vehicle rather than dissolved in it. Suspensions are also often termed 'mixtures'. As the solid is likely to separate and aggregate at the bottom of the container, it is important that the medicine is shaken before pouring a dose to ensure even distribution of the active ingredients.
- **Emulsions**: these are essentially mixtures of oil and water that are rendered homogeneous by the addition of an emulsifying agent. There can be some separation or 'creaming' of the two phases (as in milk), hence the importance of shaking the bottle before taking a dose.

The following is the procedure for taking a liquid form of medication:

1. Ideally the medicine should be taken while standing or at least sitting upright.
2. Pick up the container with the label against the palm of the hand, to protect the label from staining by any dripping medicine.
3. Shake the bottle (if necessary) and measure the dose on to the spoon.
4. Transfer to the mouth and swallow.
5. If a dose greater than 5 mL is required (e.g. 10 mL, 15 mL), repeat the process the appropriate number of times.
6. Once the dose has been taken, clean the neck of the bottle to help prevent the lid sticking. Then replace the lid.
7. If advised to take the medicine in water, transfer the measured dose to a small glass and add approximately the same amount of water to the measured dose, stir and swallow.

How to use an oral syringe
1. Shake the bottle of medicine.
2. Remove the lid and insert the bung.
3. Insert the tip of the syringe into the hole in the bung.
4. Invert the bottle.

5. Pull the plunger of the syringe back to the graduation for the dose required.
6. Turn the bottle back upright.
7. Remove the syringe from the bung, holding the barrel of the syringe rather than the plunger.
8. Gently empty the contents of the syringe into the child's mouth, inside the cheek.
9. Remove the syringe from the child's mouth.
10. Remove the bung from the bottle, clean the neck of the bottle if necessary and replace the lid.
11. Wash the bung and syringe in warm water and leave to dry. If you are giving medicine to a baby it is advised that the syringe be passed through bottle sterilising fluid as well.

Nasal drops

1. Gently blow the nose to clear the nostrils.
2. Wash hands.
3. Shake the bottle of drops. Some are suspensions and will need shaking; if applicable, this direction will be on the label.
4. Remove the lid from the bottle. If the lid includes an integral dropper draw some liquid into it.
5. Position the head as follows: the easiest position is to lie on the bed with the head hanging over the edge. Bending forward or kneeling is an alternative but maintaining the position for 2 minutes after using the drops is more difficult. Tilting the head back is not a suitable position because the drops will not cover the upper surface of the nostril.
6. Drop the required number of drops into each nostril – the intention is to spread the drop(s) evenly over the surface of the nostril. Do not allow the dropper to touch the nose.
7. Stay in position for 2 minutes to prevent the drops running out of the nose and down the back of the throat.
8. Replace the lid.

Nasal sprays

1. Gently blow nose to clear nostrils.
2. Wash hands with soapy water before using the spray.
3. Gently shake the spray. Some are suspensions and need shaking; if applicable, this direction is on the label.
4. Remove the cap from the spray.
5. Tilt head slightly forward (look down at feet).
6. Close one nostril; gently press against the side of the nose with one finger.
7. Insert tip of nasal spray into open nostril and slowly breathe in through the open nostril, and while breathing in squeeze

the spray to deliver one dose. It is important to keep the spray upright (do not sniff hard as the spray will travel straight to the back of the throat failing to deposit any medication in the nostril).

8. Remove spray from the nose and breathe out through the mouth. Tilt head backwards for about a minute to prevent the liquid spray running out of the nose.
9. Repeat in other nostril as directed.
10. Replace lid on spray.
11. Try not to blow nose for several minutes after using the spray.

Oral powders

1. Ideally powders should be taken while standing or sitting upright .
2. Open the powder carefully on a flat surface then empty the contents of the sachet either:
   - directly on to the back of the tongue and swallow with a glass of water or
   - into about a third of a tumbler-full of water, stir to disperse and swallow resulting solution/suspension.
3. Do not lie down flat for at least 2 minutes after taking the powder.

Patches

1. Freshly wash and dry the area of skin where the patch is to be applied. Do not use talc, oil, moisturisers or creams because this may prevent the patch sticking.
2. Tear open the patch package where indicated (use the fingers rather than scissors to prevent accidental damage to the patch).
3. Remove the protective backing from the patch. Try not to touch the adhesive with fingers.
4. Press the adhesive side of the patch to the prepared skin site firmly. Ensure that there is good skin contact, particularly at the edges of the patch.
5. Wash hands thoroughly with soap and water to remove any possible contamination with medicament.

Pessaries and vaginal creams

1. Wash hands with soapy water before using the pessaries/cream.
2. Remove any external foil or plastic packaging from the pessary and applicator.

3. If an applicator is provided, load the applicator as directed by the manufacturer.
4. Stand with one leg on a chair or lie down with knees bent and legs apart.
5. Press the applicator plunger to insert the pessary or cream into the vagina. If no applicator is provided, insert the pessary as high into the vagina as is comfortable by pushing gently but firmly in an upward and backward direction using the middle finger.
6. If an applicator is used wash it ready for next use.
7. Wash hands once more.

Suppositories

1. If possible go to the toilet and empty the bowels.
2. Wash hands.
3. Remove foil or plastic packaging.
4. Warm the suppository in hands to aid insertion.
5. Lie on one side with knees pulled up towards the chest or alternatively squat.
6. Gently, but firmly, insert the suppository into the rectum with a finger. Insert tapered end first. Push the suppository in as far as possible to prevent it slipping back out.
7. Lower legs and remain still for a few minutes, clenching buttocks together if necessary to retain the suppository. Unless the suppository is a laxative, avoid emptying the bowels for at least 1 hour.
8. Wash hands again.

Tablets and capsules

Types of tablet
Tablets come in various forms.

Film or sugar coated
These coatings are added by manufacturers to mask unpleasant tastes (e.g. amiodarone and metronidazole, both of which have a bitter taste) and to make the tablets easier to swallow.

Enteric coated
Enteric-coated tablets are intended to pass through the stomach unbroken and start to dissolve only when they reach the intestine. The coating may protect either the stomach from local damage by the drug (e.g. aspirin) or the drug to ensure that it is released at its intended site of action for a more local effect (e.g. bisacodyl). These tablets must therefore be swallowed whole and not crushed

or chewed because this would damage the coating and render it ineffective.

Slow-release tablets or 'SR' tablets

These tablets are designed to release their active ingredient slowly over a period of time, usually 12–24 hours. These must be swallowed whole to prevent the patient receiving a toxic dose because, instead of being absorbed over 12–24 hours, the full day's dose will be absorbed in 1–2 hours. It would also mean that there would be times during the day when the patient was receiving no medication. These tablets are also called:

- Extended release or 'XL'
- Long acting or 'LA'
- Modified release or 'MR'
- Retard
- Slow or Slo.

Effervescent, soluble or dispersible tablets

These tablets dissolve or disperse in water, making them easier to swallow in a quickly prepared liquid form. The onset of action of these tablets may be quicker than their equivalent solid ordinary tablet because the active ingredient may be more readily absorbed from the resultant liquid.

Chewable tablets

These are useful for patients who do not like to swallow tablets whole. They can be chewed and broken down in the mouth before swallowing. Commonly they are sweetened and flavoured to improve their palatability. Common examples include antacid preparations where the relatively large tablets are still more convenient than the equivalent liquid preparation.

Sublingual or buccal tablets

These are designed so that the drug itself avoids the gastrointestinal tract, therefore avoiding first-pass metabolism. It is important that the tablets are not swallowed. Sublingual tablets are designed to dissolve under the tongue and buccal tablets are designed to dissolve in the space between the gum and the cheeks or lip.

Types of capsule

Capsules are also available in two distinct forms.

Hard gelatin

These consist of two pieces that clip together. The capsule can be filled with the active drug in powder form and any necessary bulking excipient. Alternatively, controlled-release preparations can be made by giving the capsule itself an enteric coating or making pellets or beads of the active ingredient, which are then coated and packaged within the gelatin shell.

Soft gelatin
These are flexible, usually one piece and usually contain liquids, e.g. fish liver oil capsules.

The soft gelatin capsules can be coated to produce modified-release preparations or enteric-resistant coatings can be added to allow for absorption from the intestine.

Taking tablets and capsules
Taking tablets and capsules is generally a simple operation. Special consideration is given to soluble, sublingual and buccal preparations.

1. Ideally the tablets or capsules should be taken while standing or at least sitting upright.
2. Place the tablet or capsule in the mouth.
3. Swallow with the aid of a glass of water. (Plenty of water ensures that the tablet or capsule reaches the stomach and does not feel that it is 'stuck' in the throat.)
4. Do not lie down flat for at least 2 minutes.

How to take soluble tablets
1. Place the tablet or tablets into a small glassful of water.
2. Stir to dissolve the tablets.
3. Drink the resultant solution.

How to take sublingual tablets
1. Sit down.
2. Take a sip of water to moisten the mouth if it is dry.
3. Swallow or spit out the water.
4. Place the tablet under the tongue.
5. Close the mouth and do not swallow until the tablet has dissolved completely. Do not hasten the process by moving the tablet around the mouth with the tongue. Do not chew or swallow the tablet and do not eat, drink or smoke while the tablet is dissolving.
6. Do not rinse out the mouth for several minutes after the tablet has dissolved.

How to take buccal tablets
1. Sit down.
2. Take a sip of water to moisten the mouth if it is dry.
3. Swallow or spit out the water.
4. Place the tablet between the cheek and the upper or lower gum (or alternatively between the upper gum and the lip).

5. Close the mouth and do not swallow until the tablet has dissolved completely. Do not hasten the process by moving the tablet around the mouth with the tongue. Do not chew or swallow the tablet and do not eat, drink or smoke while the tablet is dissolving.
6. Do not rinse out the mouth for several minutes after the tablet has dissolved.

Topical applications

How to use an emollient cream or ointment
1. Wash area (preferably with an emollient wash) and pat dry gently with a towel (do not rub).
2. Five to ten minutes after washing apply the emollient liberally (the skin will have cooled and the water content of the skin will be highest).
3. Repeat as necessary during the day.

How to use a steroid cream or ointment
1. Wash hands.
2. Wash area (preferably with an emollient wash) and pat dry gently with a towel (do not rub).
3. Apply the cream or ointment sparingly (thinly) to the affected area.
4. Gently massage the cream or ointment into the skin.
5. After application wash hands again, unless the hands are the area being treated.

Self-assessment

Question 1
A patient calls in your pharmacy with a prescription for betamethasone valerate 0.1% cream with directions to apply to the foot twice a day. What advice would you offer this patient?

Your patient informs you that she regularly uses aqueous cream because of her dry skin and asks you the following questions:
1. **How much should I use? The doctor said something about fingertips. What did he mean?**
2. **Should this new cream be applied before or after my aqueous cream?**
3. **The doctor suggested I purchased a soap substitute. Can you recommend one?**
4. **My friend says I should wrap my feet in Clingfilm. Would this be a good idea? (If not, explain to the patient why not.)**

Question 2

A patient calls in your pharmacy with a prescription for lactulose solution with directions to take 15 mL bd. What advice would you offer this patient?

Your patient informs you that he has not taken this medication before and is quite concerned about his constipation. He asks you the following questions:

1. How long will it take to work?
2. Are there any side effects that I should know about?
3. Does it taste nice?
4. Am I likely to need to keep taking laxatives?
5. Can you advise me on how I can manage the condition without the need for regular laxatives?
6. My friend always takes Fybogel. Does it work in the same way as my medication?

Question 3

A patient calls into your pharmacy with a prescription for carteolol eyedrops 1% with instructions to use the drops twice a day. The patient has never used eyedrops before. What general advice could you offer for application of these drops?

As these drops are for the treatment of glaucoma and likely to be long term, what further information would you provide?

Your patient is grateful for your help but wondered if you could tell him how he got glaucoma because he would like to make sure that his children don't develop glaucoma when they grow up.

He is also quite concerned that he will have to stop driving as he is obviously going blind. What would you advise your patient?

Question 4

Mrs Jones calls into your pharmacy with two prescriptions, one for herself for Gaviscon Advance liquid 500 mL dose 10 mL tds pc and at bedtime, the other for her husband for 28 oxytetracycline tablets 250 mg od.

What advice would you give her? What additional advice would you need to provide if both items were for the same patient?

Question 5

Mrs Smith brings a prescription for her two-and-a-half-year-old daughter Emily. The prescription is for beclometasone inhaler (MDI 100 micrograms) one puff twice a day, a salbutamol inhaler (MDI 100 micrograms) and a spacer device.

She is concerned that her child has been diagnosed with asthma and, as she has no experience of inhalers, she needs reassurance as to how to use the inhalers and spacer device.

After you have explained the use of the inhaler to her, Mrs Smith is more confident about its use but asks you if you think it likely that Emily will grow out of asthma.

Summary

Following on from the basics of patient counselling covered in Chapter 8, this chapter summarised the key points relating to the counselling of a variety of different dosage forms.

It is important that as pharmacists and pharmacy technicians you are familiar with the points discussed in this chapter, to ensure that you can counsel patients and carers effectively in the use of different dosage forms.

Further details of how to use the different dosage forms contained within this chapter can be found in *Applied Pharmaceutical Practice* (Langley and Belcher, 2008).

chapter 10
Poisons and spirits

Overview

Upon completion of this chapter, you should be able to:

- summarise the legislation relating to the sale or supply of non-medicinal poisons that affect pharmacy, including the Poisons Act 1972 and the Poisons Rules
- review the legislation relating to the sale or supply of spirits from a pharmacy.

Introduction and overview

This chapter provides an overview of the legislation affecting the sale or supply of non-medicinal poisons and spirits from a pharmacy.

Poisons

The sale of non-medicinal poisons in England, Scotland and Wales is controlled by the Poisons Act 1972, the Poisons Rules 1982 and the Poisons List Order 1982, and amending Orders made to these statutory instruments. In Northern Ireland, non-medicinal poisons are covered by the Poisons (NI) Order 1976 and the Poisons (NI) Regulations 1983.

A non-medicinal poison is one included in the Poisons List made under the Poisons Act 1972. No matter how toxic or potent a substance may be, it will not be termed a poison unless it is included in the Poisons List. An item being listed in the Poisons List does not preclude it from also having medicinal uses. When the substance is sold for medicinal use the controls applied are those listed in the Medicines Act 1968; it is only when they are sold for non-medicinal purposes that they are subject to the Poisons Act.

The Poisons List

The Poisons List is the list of substances that are classed as poisons under the Poisons Act and set out in the Poisons List Order. The list is divided into two parts:

- **Part I**: these are non-medicinal poisons that may be sold only by persons lawfully conducting a retail pharmacy business. In other words they can be sold only from a registered pharmacy. The sale must be either by the pharmacist or under the supervision of a pharmacist.

KeyPoints

The Poisons List is divided into two parts:

Part I: these are non-medicinal poisons that may only be sold by persons lawfully conducting a retail pharmacy business

Part II: these are non-medicinal poisons that may only be sold by persons lawfully conducting a retail pharmacy business or a person (or nominated deputy/deputies) who is included on a local authority's list of persons entitled to sell non-medicinal poisons in Part II of the list.

- **Part II**: these are non-medicinal poisons that may be sold only by persons lawfully conducting a retail pharmacy business or a person who is included on a local authority's list of persons entitled to sell non-medicinal poisons in Part II of the list (known as a 'listed seller'). The Part II list contains non-medicinal poisons that are in common usage for non-medicinal purposes.

Inclusion on the list of sellers is by application and the local authority can refuse permission if they believe that a person is unfit. Similarly a person can be deleted from the list for non-payment of a retention fee or following a conviction that would make the person unfit to sell poisons. Each listed seller may nominate one or two deputies who may effect the sale of Schedule 1 poisons.

The Poisons Rules

The Poisons Rules are the detailed legislation of the Poisons Act; they outline rules regarding transport and containers, record keeping and storage. The Rules ensure the safe distribution and storage of poisons. In addition the Rules may either place additional controls on substances or alternatively relax some controls where deemed necessary through schedules.

There were originally 12 schedules. Schedules 2, 3, 6 and 7 were deleted by the Poisons Rules Amendment Order in 1985. The function of the remaining eight schedules is detailed below.

Schedule 1

Below is a list of substances to which special restrictions apply with regard to sale, storage and the keeping of records.

Conditions of sale – knowledge of the purchaser

- A person to whom the poison may properly be sold. The purchaser is either known to be so by the seller or a pharmacist on the premises or the purchaser must produce a certificate stating that he or she is a person who may be supplied.
- The certificate is a declaration made by a householder (see Schedule 10 below) and if the householder is unknown to the seller it must also be endorsed by a police officer in charge of a police station. Please note that the police endorse the good character of the householder, who may not necessarily be the purchaser. The seller must retain the certificate for 2 years from the date of supply.

Storage
- Must be stored separately from other items, e.g. in a cupboard or drawer specifically for that purpose or in a separate part of the premises where customers have no access or on a shelf reserved for poisons storage that has no food stored below it.
- If used in agriculture/horticulture/forestry:
  - store separate from food products (i.e. not in part of the premises where food is kept)
  - if stored in a drawer or cupboard or on a shelf it must be reserved solely for the storage of poisons.

Labels and containers
- The labelling of poisons and the containers used are subject to the CHIP (Chemicals (Hazard Information and Packaging for Supply) Regulations.

Records
- The purchaser must sign the completed poisons register as outlined in Schedule 11.
- Signed orders apply to sales for purpose of trade, business or profession. The signed order replaces the signature in the poisons register. The order must be given before the sale and state:
  - name and address of the purchaser
  - nature of trade, business or profession
  - purpose for which poison is required
  - total quantities of poison to be supplied
  - the date (although it is not a legal requirement, the Home Office has indicated that a date should be present on a signed order for a non-medicinal poison).
- The seller must be satisfied that the signature is correct, the person does carry out that occupation and the poison is reasonably needed for that occupation.
- The poisons register must be retained for 2 years from the last entry/record.

Emergency supply
- In an emergency, a Schedule 1 poison may be supplied on an undertaking that a signed order will be supplied within 72 hours. You must be satisfied that:
  - there is an emergency
  - an order cannot be produced.
- It would be prudent to make an emergency supply only to someone known to you personally.

Relaxation of conditions of sale
The conditions for sale of Schedule 1 poisons are relaxed in certain circumstances, when 'knowledge of the purchaser by the

seller' is interpreted as personal knowledge of the purchaser by the seller and the seller knows that the purchaser is a person to whom the poison may properly be sold. This relaxation is applied to the following:

- Sales of Part II Schedule 1 poisons by listed sellers
- Provision of commercial samples of Schedule 1 poisons
- Sales of Schedule 1 poisons exempted under Section 4 of the Act
- Schedule 1 poisons are exempt from the conditions of sale and record keeping if the poison is to be exported to a purchaser outside the UK, or if the sale is made by a manufacturer or wholesaler to a person who is carrying on a business in the course of which poisons are sold or regularly used in the manufacture of other articles, and the seller is satisfied that the purchaser is a person who requires the article for use in his or her business.

Schedule 4
This is a list of substances that are exempt from poison controls. There are two groups:

- Group I: this consists of articles containing poisons that are totally exempt from poisons law.
- Group II: this lists exemptions for certain poisons when they are in specified articles or substances.

Schedule 5
Schedule 5 lists those Part II poisons that may be sold only by listed sellers in certain forms. Schedule 5 is divided into two parts: Parts A and B. In any other circumstances, the sale of Schedule 5 poisons is restricted to pharmacies.

Schedule 8
This outlines the detail required in the form for application for inclusion in the local authority's list of sellers of Part II poisons.

Schedule 9
This outlines the detail required in the form for the local authority's list of sellers of Part II poisons.

Schedule 10
This outlines the details to be entered on a certificate for the purchase of a poison.

Schedule 11
This specifies the details that need to be recorded in the poisons book on sale of a Schedule 1 poison.

Schedule 12
This applies to restrictions of the sale and supply of strychnine and other substances and the forms of authority required for certain of these poisons. Schedule 12 places further controls on some Schedule 1 poisons.

Section 4 Exemptions
Section 4 of the Poisons Act 1972 lists circumstances when poisons may be sold by individuals who are neither non-pharmacists nor listed sellers. Exemptions include:
- wholesale dealing
- export from the UK
- sale to a doctor, dentist or vet for professional purposes
- sale for use in a hospital or similar institution
- sale by wholesale:
  - to a government department
  - for education or research
  - to enable employers to meet any statutory obligation with respect to medical treatment of employees
  - to a person requiring the substance for trade, business or profession.

Spirits

In England and Wales the main legislation controlling sale and supply of alcohol is:
- Customs and Excise Management Act 1979
- Alcohol Liquor Duties Act 1979
- Denatured Alcohol Regulations 2005.

The legislation relating to spirits within Scotland has historically been different and was controlled by the Methylated Spirits (Sale by Retail) (Scotland) Act 1937. Many of the requirements of the 1937 Act were removed by the Deregulated Methylated Spirits (Sale by Retail) (Scotland) Order 1988. However, section 1(2), which prohibits the sale of methylated spirits to any person under the age of 14, still applies. In addition, the Denatured Alcohol Regulations 2005 also apply in Scotland.

Definition of spirits
The term 'spirits' refers to ethyl alcohol and includes all liquor mixed with spirits and all mixtures, compounds or preparations made with spirits. It does not, however, include denatured alcohol.

Duty is payable on all alcohol imported into the UK and excise duty is levied on all alcohol distilled in the UK.

In order to sell alcohol in the UK a justice's licence is required. This normally applies to public houses, off-licences, supermarkets, etc. A pharmacy would need a licence in order to retail an alcoholic tonic wine but does not need a licence in order to supply or manufacture medicines containing alcohol. A pharmacy would also be exempt from the requirement to hold a licence if selling alcohol to a trader for purposes of trade.

Pharmacists are mainly concerned with the dispensing of alcohol. The *Drug Tariff* states:

> Where Alcohol (96%), or Rectified Spirit (Ethanol 90%), or any other of the dilute Ethanols is prescribed as an ingredient of a medicine for internal use, the price of the duty paid to Customs and Excise will be allowed, unless the contractor endorses the prescription form 'rebate claimed'.

In other words the duty that we have to pay if we include a spirit in a medicine on an NHS prescription has been returned to us via the reimbursement that we receive as stated in the *Drug Tariff*. The use of alcohol in mixtures prepared extemporaneously has declined with the advent of products that can now more effectively control pain. *Brompton cocktail* was used to treat pain in terminal cancer patients. It consisted of morphine and cocaine and was made up in a vehicle consisting of alcohol, syrup and chloroform water. It was common practice to ask the patient which spirit they preferred, e.g. whisky, brandy, gin or rum.

Denatured alcohol

Denatured alcohol is controlled by Alcohol Liquor Duties Act 1979 and Denatured Alcohol Regulations 2005. There are three types of denatured alcohol, but in pharmacy we mainly encounter two types, namely completely denatured alcohol (CDA), which was formerly known as mineralised methylated spirits (MMS), and industrial denatured alcohol (IDA), formerly known as industrial methylated spirit (IMS). The third, less commonly encountered denatured alcohol is trade-specific denatured alcohol (TSDA). The formulae for these denatured alcohols render them unfit for human consumption (see the current edition of *Medicines, Ethics and Practice: A guide for pharmacists and pharmacy technicians* (see Bibliography) for details of formulae for denaturing or HM Customs and Excise notice 473 [2005]).

For a pharmacy to receive IDA or TSDA for sale or use within the pharmacy, it must apply to the HM Revenue and Customs National Registration Unit in order to gain authority to receive. Authorisation must be obtained before a supply of IDA or TSDA can be made. Once authorisation has been granted, a copy of the authorisation must be sent to the supplier and then a supply can be made.

A community pharmacist is then authorised to dispense IDA on a prescription either alone or as an ingredient for an item for external use only, such as a liniment or lotion (this could be for human or animal use). IDA may also be sold by the community pharmacist but only for medical or scientific purposes; again the purchaser would need to have authorisation and a copy of this authorisation would need to be in the pharmacist's possession. It should be noted that the supply can be made only for the use indicated on the user's authorisation and no other. When labelled for a dispensed item the label must clearly state 'For external use only' and also *British National Formulary* caution 15 'Caution flammable: keep away from fire or flames'. In the case of labelling for sale this is as outlined in the CHIP regulations.

Conditions are attached to the authority to receive IDA or TSDA and include the following:

- **Storage**: an undertaking must be made that the IDA or TSDA will be stored under lock and key and under the pharmacist's personal control or under the control of an authorised deputy.
- **Use**: this must be only as laid out in the authorisation.
- **Supply**: only approved formulations of alcohol can be supplied and if this is not on a prescription a written statement from the authorised user must be obtained or, in the case of a medical practitioner, a written order.
- **Close of business**: should a business close, the authorisation to possess denatured alcohol would be withdrawn. The National Advice Centre of HM Revenue and Customs should be contacted to arrange how stocks should be disposed of and over what period of time. Once the stock has been cleared the National Registration Unit should be informed in order to cancel the authorisation.
- When IDA or TSDA is received a record of the amount of IDA or TSDA received must be made and a copy of the supplier's delivery note must be signed and returned to the supplier; a second copy must be retained on the premises as an additional record of the supply.

The quantity of CDA that can be supplied has no restriction in the UK; there are also no restrictions on its use (it is commonly used in 'meths burners', e.g. in fondue sets). It is supplied free from duty. IDA and TSDA have more restrictions and may be supplied in quantities less than 20 litres, only to authorised users, but there is no restriction on the amount that can be supplied to a medical practitioner on a written order.

All records must show the amount of IDA or TSDA received and supplied and any excess or deficiency in the balance must be accounted for because, if it has been found to be supplied for an unauthorised use, a demand may be issued by HM Customs and Excise for the duty payable on the alcohol in the missing amount.

Records of IDA and TSDA

Generally, records must be kept as set out in Notice 206 Revenue Traders Accounts and Records. Specifically:

- a stock account of all the spirits received and used
- such other records as are either specified in the letter of authority, or are necessary to establish that the spirits have been put to the authorised use.

Records must also be kept of all the checks carried out on receipts, storage and use of the spirits. Normal business records may be used for these purposes provided that there is a clear audit trail from receipt to final disposal. Records must be kept up to date. In addition:

- stock accounts should be balanced at the intervals as required by the letter of authority. The physical stock should be checked and the result noted in the account
- any apparent discrepancies should be investigated promptly, and any that cannot be resolved should be reported to the local office immediately.

Records must be kept for at least 6 years.

Self-assessment

For questions 1–9, **ONE** or **MORE** of the responses/statements is/are correct. Decide which of the responses/statements is/are correct and then choose:

A   If statements 1, 2 and 3 are all correct
B   If statements 1 and 2 are correct and statement 3 is incorrect
C   If statements 2 and 3 are correct and statement 1 is incorrect
D   If statement 1 is correct and statements 2 and 3 are incorrect
E   If statement 3 is correct and statements 1 and 2 are incorrect

Question 1

The sale of non-medicinal poisons in England, Scotland and Wales is controlled by:

1. **The Pharmacy and Poisons Act 1933**
2. **The Medicines Act 1968**
3. **The Poisons Act 1972**

Question 2

Concerning the sale of alcohol in England and Wales:

1. **The sale and supply of products containing ethyl alcohol (ethanol) are controlled ONLY by the Alcohol Liquor Duties Act 1979.**

2. The sale and supply of completely denatured alcohol (CDA) are controlled ONLY by the Denatured Alcohol Regulations 2005.
3. The sale and supply of industrial denatured alcohol (IDA) are controlled by the Alcohol Liquor Duties Act 1979 and Denatured Alcohol Regulations 2005.

Question 3

Which of the following statements concerning poisons is/are true?
1. The Poisons Board or advisory committee must include at least five people appointed by the RPSGB.
2. All non-medicinal poisons must be labelled with the word 'Poison' for the purpose of the Poisons Act 1972.
3. The Poisons Act 1972 applies in England, Scotland, Wales and Northern Ireland.

Question 4

Which of the following statements concerning non-medicinal poisons is/are correct?
1. A Part II non-medicinal poison may be sold ONLY by a person listed with the local authority.
2. Some substances that are listed as poisons are also included in some medicinal products. These substances and products containing these substances are controlled by both the Medicines Act 1968 and the Poisons Act 1972.
3. A non-medicinal poison is defined as a substance listed in Part I or II of the Poisons List; other substances regardless of toxicity are not poisons.

Question 5

Which of the following statements with regard to the Poisons Act 1972 is/are true?
1. If a person requesting to purchase a Schedule 1 poison for use in their business provides a written order, there is no legal requirement for a poison register entry to be made.
2. Poisons listed in Part 1 of the Poisons List may be sold ONLY from registered pharmacies.
3. Schedule I of the Poisons Rules may be applied to both Part I and Part II poisons.

Question 6

In the case of a signed order for a Schedule 1, Part I poison, which of the following are **LEGALLY** required?
1. Name and address of purchaser
2. Nature of the trade, business or profession
3. The date

Question 7

With regard to the supply and storage of industrial denatured alcohol which of the following statements is/are correct?

1. **Stocks must be kept in locked containers.**
2. **Medicinal products containing IDA must be labelled 'For external use only' and 'Caution flammable: keep away from fire or flame'.**
3. **The maximum amount of IDA that can be supplied on an NHS prescription is 500 mL.**

Question 8

With regard to the supply of spirits from a registered pharmacy, which of the following statements is/are correct?

1. **Any pharmacy wishing to sell alcoholic tonic wine must hold a justice's licence.**
2. **Pharmacists are permitted to dispense medicines containing spirits such as brandy and whisky.**
3. **If a spirit is supplied on NHS prescription as an ingredient of a dispensed medicine, the duty paid will be returned via the reimbursement received from the PPD (or equivalent).**

Question 9

Nicotine can be considered a medicinal product (general sale list or GSL) and also in other circumstances a Part II poison. When selling nicotine replacement patches over the counter the legislation that covers the sale is:

1. **The Medicines Act 1968**
2. **The Poisons Act 1972**
3. **Both the Poisons Act 1972 and the Medicines Act 1968.**

Summary

This chapter has summarised the key points of the regulations for the sale and supply of both poisons and spirits that pharmacists and pharmacy technicians should be aware of. Many pharmacists in daily practice may never supply poisons or spirits; however, it is possible that requests will be made from time to time. Therefore, it is important that pharmacists and pharmacy technicians are familiar with the key points.

Further and more detailed information on the sale and supply of poisons and spirits can be found in *Applied Pharmaceutical Practice* (Langley and Belcher, 2008), the current edition of *Medicines, Ethics and Practice: A guide for pharmacists and pharmacy technicians* (see Bibliography) and *Dale and Appelbe's Pharmacy Law and Ethics* (Appelbe and Wingfield, 2005).

Answers to self-assessment

Chapter 1

Question 1
Answer: C

Statements 2 and 3 are correct and statement 1 is incorrect.

POMs may be sold in particular circumstances, e.g. in an emergency supply at the request of a patient or when a prescription-only medicine (POM) is sold to a patient on production of a private (non-NHS) prescription form (see Chapter 5).

Question 2
Answer: E

Statement 3 is correct and statements 1 and 2 are incorrect.

Although in practice all may be treated as P medicines, legally there is a subtle difference between supervision and personal control.

Question 3
Answer: A

Statements 1, 2 and 3 are all correct.

Question 4
Answer: B

Statements 1 and 2 are correct and statement 3 is incorrect.

Question 5
Answer: C

Statements 2 and 3 are correct and statement 1 is incorrect.

Only (1) can be a general sale list (GSL) medicine.

Question 6
Answer: B

Statements 1 and 2 are correct and statement 3 is incorrect.

Anusol suppositories are the only GSL medicine in the list.

Question 7
Answer: D

Statement 1 is correct and statements 2 and 3 are incorrect.

Question 8
Answer: B

Counter prescribing.

Question 9
Answer: E
100 paracetamol tablets 500 mg.

Question 10
Answer: D
The maximum single dose is 500 mg.
Naproxen can be sold to women between the ages of 15 and 50; max. pack size is 3 days' supply, i.e. 9 × 250 mg tabs; the max. daily dose is 750 mg and it is indicated for the treatment of dysmenorrhoea.

Question 11
Answer: C
It is indicated to treat reactions to insect bites and stings.
Only cream is licensed for GSL sale, the maximum pack size is 10 g (15 g is pharmacy or P medicine); its use is restricted to adults and children over 10 years, and the maximum treatment is 3 days.

Question 12
Answer: B
It is not a legal requirement for 64 paracetamol tablets to be sold by, or under the supervision of, a pharmacist.
The sale of 16–32 paracetamol tablets is classified as GSL but the limit to quantities for sale through pharmacies is set at 100 at one time. A P medicine is defined as being a medicine that is not a GSL or POM so there is no definitive list. Hypromellose eye drops are a P medicine, so cannot be sold. P medicines may be sold only from registered premises; the presence of a pharmacist is not sufficient to allow the sale through unregistered premises. Homeopathic medicines are subject to the same exemptions as traditional medicines, so injections cannot be classified as GSL medicines, nor can eyedrops, eye ointments, anthelmintics, etc.

Chapter 2

Question 1
Answer: D
Statement 1 is correct and statements 2 and 3 are incorrect.
The name and address of the prescriber and the patient's home address are found on the front of an FP10. If the patient's representative is claiming exemption on behalf of the patient, the name and address of the representative, along with their signature, must be provided on the reverse of the prescription form.

Question 2
Answer: B
Statements 1 and 2 are correct and statement 3 is incorrect.
FP10MDA-SS is a computer-generated instalment prescription, FP10MDA-S is a handwritten instalment prescription and FP10SS is a standard computer-generated NHS prescription form.

Question 3
Answer: B
Statements 1 and 2 are correct and statement 3 is incorrect.
This is the list of foods, cosmetics, etc., approved for specific medical conditions. The pharmacist will always receive payment for the supply but, in the absence of suitable endorsement by the prescriber, the prescriber may be asked to justify the use of the item and ultimately asked to pay for the item by the Prescription Pricing Division (PPD or equivalent). Pharmacists are not allowed to add the ACBS endorsement. If it is omitted from the prescription, the prescriber would normally be contacted and asked to add the necessary endorsement.

Question 4
Answer: B
Statements 1 and 2 are correct and statement 3 is incorrect.
The prescriber is not legally required to add directions to the patient on a prescription. The pharmacist should always check that the patient has these instructions; if not he or she should contact the prescriber to verify the instructions or provide suitable instructions him- or herself.

Question 5
Answer: C
It is a legal requirement that all prescriptions for a POM contain an appropriate date.
The age or date of birth of a patient is legally required only if the patient is under 12 years of age. Instalment prescribing is not allowed on an FP10NC; an FP10MDA-S would be the equivalent instalment prescription but very few items can be prescribed in instalments on NHS prescriptions. An appropriate date is legally required on an NHS prescription. Doctors must issue separate FP10 (or equivalent) prescription forms for each patient. Not all chemical reagents are allowed on FP10 (or equivalent) prescription forms; a list of those allowed can be found in the *Drug Tariff for England and Wales*, Part IXR (or equivalent).

Question 6
Answer: D
When writing NHS prescriptions a practitioner may use carbon paper to make a number of copies; each will be valid provided that the prescriber signs each copy of the prescription in indelible ink. Community practitioner nurse prescribers and dentists may prescribe only items listed in their formularies. NHS prescription forms can be dispensed only on one occasion and pharmacist independent prescribers cannot prescribe any licensed POM because they are at present unable to prescribe controlled drugs listed within Schedule 2.

Question 7
Answer: C
Two charges.
There is one charge for the phenoxymethylpenicillin antibiotic tablets and one for the warfarin tablets (as they are different strengths of the same drug in the same form).

Question 8
Answer: D
Three charges.
In this case there would be two charges on the first prescription and one on the second. Each item is a prescription, but the items when split over two forms must be dealt with as two independent events because the prescriptions need not be presented at the same time.

Question 9
Answer: C
Two charges.
There is a charge for each of the inhalers; however, there is no charge for the oral contraceptive (Microgynon 30).

Question 10
Answer: C
Two charges.
There is a charge for each item because, although they are the same drug, they are in different forms (capsules and tablets), so there is a charge for each form.

Question 11
Answer: C
Two charges.
This is because there are two different types of tablet contained within the packaging. The package is designed for ease of use by the patient; the items could be prescribed separately (14 tablets of conjugated oestrogens 625 micrograms and 14 tablets of conjugated oestrogens and medroxyprogesterone acetate 10 mg).

Question 12
Answer: B
One charge.
This is because, unlike the example in Question 11, all the tablets in this pack are identical.

Question 13
Answer: E
Four charges.
Remember that each individual piece of hosiery attracts a charge (in this case the pair of anklets would attract two charges).

Question 14
Answer: C
Two charges.
There is a charge for each product, not individual charges for the flavours.

Chapter 3

Question 1

1. **Identity of order.**
   NHS prescription (FP10SS).
2. **Prescriber.**
   Doctor (general practitioner).
3. **Legally written?**
   Yes.
4. **Clinical check (complete Table 11.1).**

Table 11.1

Drug	Indications	Dose check	Reference
Senna	Constipation	Two to four tablets usually at night: initial dose should be low, then gradually increased	*British National Formulary*, 56th edn, section 1.6.4
Digoxin	Heart failure	Maintenance 62.5–500 micrograms daily Usual dose 125–250 micrograms daily (lower dose may be appropriate in elderly people)	*British National Formulary*, 56th edn, section 2.1

5. **Interactions**
   The drugs on the prescription do not interact. However, it would also be advisable for the pharmacist or pharmacy technician to check the patient's medication record (PMR) for any concurrent medication that could cause an interaction.
6. **Suitability for patient**
   The Senokot is safe and suitable for the patient, but the digoxin is not safe or suitable. First, the strength of the digoxin should be micrograms not milligrams and a once-daily dose would be more suitable. The patient is elderly so a lower dose (perhaps 125 micrograms daily) should be considered.
7. **Item(s) allowable on the NHS**
   Senokot is not allowed on NHS FP10 prescription (see *Drug Tariff for England and Wales*, section XVIIIA). Need to ask prescriber to change the prescription to generic senna tablets which are allowed to be prescribed on FP10. The directions remain the same.
8. **Records to be made (including copies of the record[s])**
   Make a note of the interventions on a clinical intervention form. Both the change to one digoxin 125 microgram tablet od and the change to generic senna tablets must be noted.
9. **Process prescription (including example of label[s])**
   - Prepare labels.
   - Check appendix 9 of the *British National Formulary* for supplementary labelling requirements (there are none).
   - Select tablets from shelf, remembering to check expiry dates.

- Perform final check of items, labels and prescription form.
- Pack in a suitable bag ready to give to patient/patient's representative.

Labels (we have assumed that the name and address of the pharmacy and the words 'Keep out of the reach and sight of children' are pre-printed on the label) (Figure 11.1).

Figure 11.1

Digoxin 125 microgram tablets	5
Take ONE tablet every morning.	
Ada Davies	Date of dispensing

Senna tablets	20
Take TWO tablets when required.	
Ada Davies	Date of dispensing

10. Endorse prescription

Stamp with pharmacy stamp to indicate completion.

11. Destination of paperwork

Send to the PPD at the end of the month.

12. Identity check/counselling

- Check patient's name and address.
- Explain change in medication without alarming the patient.
- Advise patient to take one digoxin tablet each day.
- It is important to take them regularly and not to stop taking them unless advised to do so by the doctor.
- It may help to try to take them at the same time each day.
- Take two senna tablets at night when required.
- Advise that it may take 8–12 hours to have an effect.
- There may be some slight 'tummy' pain but generally this goes away quite quickly.
- To prevent constipation eat plenty of fibre – fruit and vegetables, bran, drink plenty of fluid and if possible take some exercise, e.g. gentle walking.
- Draw patient's attention to the patient information leaflet (PIL) and ask if she has any questions.

Question 2

1. Identity of order

NHS prescription (FP10SS).

2. Prescriber

Doctor (GP).

3. Legally written?

Yes.

4. Clinical check (complete Table 11.2).

Table 11.2

Drug	Indications	Dose check	Reference
Glyceryl trinitrate sublingual	Treatment of angina	0.3–1 mg sublingually, repeated when required	*British National Formulary*, 56th edn, section 2.6.1
Glyceryl trinitrate patches	Prophylaxis of angina	One '5' or '10' patch every 24 h	*British National Formulary*, 56th edn, section 2.6.1
Naproxen	Pain and inflammation in rheumatic disease	0.5–1 g daily in one to two divided doses	*British National Formulary*, 56th edn, section 10.1.1
Paracetamol	Mild-to-moderate pain, pyrexia	0.5–1 g every 4–6 h to a max. of 4 g in 24 h	*British National Formulary*, 56th edn, section 4.7

5. Interactions

The drugs on the prescription do not interact. However, it would also be advisable for the pharmacist or pharmacy technician to check the PMR for any concurrent medication that could cause an interaction.

6. Suitability for patient

The glyceryl trinitrate prescribed is safe and suitable for a patient of this age and the dose ordered on the prescription is within the recommended dose limits; however, the use of NSAIDs (non-steroidal anti-inflammatory drugs) in elderly people is not recommended and consideration should be given to requesting the doctor to change to paracetamol (see *British National Formulary*, 56th edn, 'Prescribing for the elderly'). Suggest 2 qds, mitte 50, especially as the PMR indicated that the item has not been prescribed previously.

7. Item(s) allowable on the NHS

Yes (see *Drug Tariff*).

8. Records to be made (including copies of the record[s])

Make a note of the intervention on a clinical intervention form.

9. Process prescription (including example of label[s])

- Prepare a label for each product.
- Check appendix 9 of the *British National Formulary* for supplementary labelling requirements:

  Paracetamol: *British National Formulary* label numbers 29 (Do not take more than 2 at any one time. Do not take more than 8 in 24 hours.) and 30 (Do not take with any other paracetamol products.).
  Glyceryl trinitrate tablets: *British National Formulary* label number 16 (Allow to dissolve under the tongue. Do not transfer from this container. Keep tightly closed. Discard 8 weeks after opening.).
  Glyceryl trinitrate patches: no additional *British National Formulary* labels.

- Glyceryl trinitrate tablets 500 micrograms must be supplied in original glass container with foil-lined lid with no cotton wool or wadding.

- Glyceryl trinitrate 10 patches, the pack size is 28 (brand Deponit or Transiderm-Nitro; best to check if patient has had either before as often prefer to stick with brand previously used).
- Select items from shelf, remembering to check expiry dates.
- Perform final check of items, labels and prescription form.
- Pack in a suitable bag ready to give to patient/patient's representative.

Labels (we have assumed that the name and address of the pharmacy and the words 'Keep out of the reach and sight of children' are pre-printed on the label.) (Figure 11.2)

Figure 11.2

Glyceryl Trinitrate Tablets 500 mcg	100
Allow one to dissolve under the tongue when required.	
Do not transfer from this container.	
Keep tightly closed.	
Discard 8 weeks after opening.	
Mr Henry Humphries	Date of dispensing

Glyceryl Trinitrate Patches 10	28
Apply one patch every morning.	
For external use only.	
Read the leaflet provided with this medication.	
Mr Henry Humphries	Date of dispensing

Paracetamol Tablets 500 mg	50
Take TWO tablets FOUR times a day.	
Do not take more than 2 at any one time or 8 in 24 hours.	
Do not take with other paracetamol products.	
Mr Henry Humphries	Date of dispensing

10. Endorse prescription

Stamp with pharmacy stamp to indicate completion.

11. Destination of paperwork

Send to the PPD at the end of the month.

12. Identity check/counselling

- Check patient's name and address.
- Explain change in medication to patient without alarming him.
- Ensure that the patient knows how to take the glyceryl trinitrate tablets. Explain that they are designed so that the drug itself avoids the gastrointestinal tract. It is therefore important that the tablets are not swallowed. Sublingual tablets are designed to dissolve under the tongue.
- Ensure that the patient knows how to apply the patches:

    Apply one patch each morning. Freshly wash and dry the area of skin where the patch is to be applied. Do not use talc, oil, moisturisers or creams as this may prevent the patch sticking.

    Tear open the patch package where indicated (use the fingers rather than scissors to prevent accidental damage to the patch).

    Remove the protective backing from the patch. Try not to touch the adhesive with fingers.

    Press the adhesive side of the patch to the prepared skin site firmly. Ensure that there is good skin contact, particularly at the edges of the patch.

Wash hands thoroughly with soap and water to remove any possible contamination with medicament.

Glyceryl trinitrate patches for angina should be applied to chest or upper arm.

Do not apply to the same site each day as irritation can occur.

Directions are included in the PIL.

- Two paracetamol tablets should be taken four times a day. It is important not to take more than the recommended dosage and not to take any other paracetamol-containing medicines (e.g. any cold and flu remedies that contain paracetamol).
- Draw patient's attention to the PILs and ask if he has any questions.

Question 3

1. **Identity of order**
   NHS prescription (FP10SS).
2. **Prescriber**
   Doctor (GP).
3. **Legally written?**
   No. The doctor failed to sign the prescription.
   The prescription will need to be returned to the prescriber for addition of signature before dispensing. The size of crêpe bandage needs to be specified (in this case for sprained ankle a 7.5 cm crepe bandage would be sensible).
4. **Clinical check (complete Table 11.3).**

Table 11.3

Drug	Indications	Dose check	Reference
Crepe bandage	Light support system for strains, sprains and compression; over paste bandages for varicose veins	Sizes available 5 cm, 7.5 cm, 10 cm and 15 cm × 4.5 m	*British National Formulary*, 56th edn, section A8.2.4

5. **Interactions**
   None.
6. **Suitability for patient**
   On questioning patient has sprained ankle.
7. **Item(s) allowable on the NHS**
   Yes (see *Drug Tariff*).
8. **Records to be made (including copies of the record[s])**
   Make a note of the intervention on a clinical intervention form.
9. **Process prescription**
   - As the bandages are non-medicated they do not require a label.
   - Perform final check of item and prescription.
   - Pack in a suitable bag ready to give to the patient or patient's representative.
10. **Endorse prescription**
    Stamp with pharmacy stamp to indicate completion.

11. Destination of paperwork

Send to the PPD at the end of the month.

12. Identity check/counselling

- Check patient's name and address.
- Ensure that he knows how to apply the bandage.
- Keep the injured part of the body supported in the position that it will be in when the bandage is on.
- After you have put the bandage on, secure the end by folding it over and tying a knot in the end; you can also use a safety pin, adhesive (sticky) tape or bandage clip.
- As soon as you have put the bandage on, check if the bandage feels too tight and check the circulation by pressing a nail or a piece of skin until it turns pale. If the colour does not return straight away the bandage may be too tight, so you should loosen it. Limbs can swell up after an injury so check the circulation after the bandage has been applied.

Question 4

1. **Identity of order**

   NHS prescription (FP10SS).

2. **Prescriber**

   Doctor (GP).

3. **Legally written?**

   No. Date omitted. Return prescription form to prescriber for addition.

4. **Clinical check (complete Table 11.4).**

Table 11.4

Drug	Indications	Dose check	Reference
Amiodarone	Treatment of arrhythmias	200 mg tds for 1 week, reduced to 200 bd for a further week; maintenance usually 200 mg daily	*British National Formulary*, 56th edn, section 2.3.2
SpectraBan lotion	Skin protection against UVA and UVB photodermatoses	Apply thickly and frequently (approximately every 2 h)	*British National Formulary*, 56th edn, section 13.8.1

5. **Interactions**

   The drugs on the prescription do not interact. However, it would also be advisable for the pharmacist or pharmacy technician to check the PMR for any concurrent medication that could cause an interaction. Amiodarone has been known to interact with grapefruit juice.

6. **Suitability for patient**

   The amiodarone dose is higher than the maintenance dose for arrhythmias so need to check that it is the second week of treatment and therefore safe and suitable for the patient. The SpectraBan Ultra is a sunblock prescribed to prevent skin damage that may occur because amiodarone can sensitise the skin and photodermatoses are a common side effect.

7. **Item(s) allowable on the NHS**

Yes (see *Drug Tariff for England and Wales*, Part XV [Borderline substances]). The prescription needs to be returned to the prescriber for the addition of ACBS endorsement to the SpectraBan Ultra so that it will be passed for payment by the PPD. The endorsement shows that the item has been prescribed in accordance with the recommendations laid down by the Advisory Committee.

8. **Records to be made (including copies of the record[s])**

Make a note of the intervention on a clinical intervention form (both the ACBS and date intervention and the check that the treatment was for the second week of therapy with amiodarone).

9. **Process prescription (including example of label[s])**
    - Prepare a label for each product.
    - Check appendix 9 of the *British National Formulary* for supplementary labelling requirements:
        Amiodarone: *British National Formulary* label number 11 (Avoid exposure of skin to direct sunlight or sunlamps.).
        SpectraBan Ultra: no additional *British National Formulary* labels.
    - Select items from shelf, remembering to check expiry dates.
    - Perform final check of items, labels and prescription form.
    - Pack in a suitable bag ready to give to patient.

Labels (we have assumed that the name and address of the pharmacy and the words 'Keep out of the reach and sight of children' are pre-printed on the label.) (Figure 11.3).

Amiodarone Tablets 200 mg   14
Take ONE tablet TWICE a day.
Avoide Exposure of skin to direct sunlight or sun lamps.
Mr Christopher Benson   Date of dispensing

Figure 11.3

SpectraBan Ultra SPF 28 Lotion   150 ml
Apply as directed.
For external use only.
Mr Christopher Benson   Date of dispensing

10. **Endorse prescription**

Stamp with pharmacy stamp to indicate completion.

11. **Destination of paperwork**

Send to the PPD at the end of the month.

12. **Identity check/counselling**
     - Check patient's name and address.
     - Check that this is the second week of therapy with amiodarone. Advise that patient should take one tablet twice daily and the tablets be swallowed whole. Try to take at the same times each day to avoid missing any doses.
     - Amiodarone can affect your eyes, making it difficult to drive at night or in poor visibility because the headlights dazzle.

- It is advisable to avoid grapefruit juice when taking amiodarone.
- The SpectraBan is a sunblock to help prevent any light sensitivity reactions associated with the use of amiodarone. It needs to be applied liberally; a single application may be sufficient but reapplication is advised to ensure total block.
- Draw patient's attention to the PIL and ask if he has any questions.

Chapter 4

Question 1

1. **Identity of order**
   Inpatient drug chart.
2. **Prescriber**
   Doctor (hospital doctor).
3. **Legally written?**
   Yes.
4. **Clinical check (complete Table 11.5)**

Table 11.5

Drug	Indications	Dose check	Reference
Digoxin	Heart failure, supraventricular arrhythmias	Maintenance, usual range 125–250 micrograms daily	British National Formulary, 56th edn, section 2.1.1
Ciprofloxacin	Infections	Respiratory tract infections, 250–750 mg twice daily	British National Formulary, 56th edn, section 5.1.12

5. **Interactions**
   There is no interaction between the digoxin tablets and the ciprofloxacin tablets. In addition, the ward pharmacist should check the other sections of the patient's inpatient drug chart for any additional concurrent medication that could cause an interaction. In this case, the other sections of the patient's inpatient drug chart did not contain the details of any other medication.
6. **Suitability for patient**
   The item prescribed is safe and suitable for an adult patient and the dose ordered on the prescription is within the recommended dose limits.
   The ward pharmacist can order the ciprofloxacin from the pharmacy via an inpatient order as shown in Figure 11.4.
7. **Records to be made (including copies of the record[s])**
   None.
8. **Process prescription (including example of label[s])**
   The inpatient order would be sent to the pharmacy and the pharmacy technician would dispense 10 ciprofloxacin 250 mg tablets (remembering to check the expiry date). After checking, this would be sent to the ward, labelled with the patient's name. As the medication will be administered by

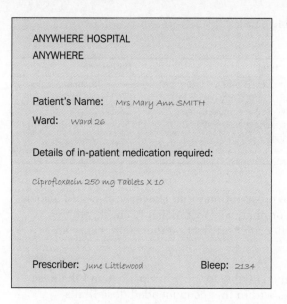

Figure 11.4

ANYWHERE HOSPITAL
ANYWHERE

Patient's Name: Mrs Mary Ann SMITH

Ward: Ward 26

Details of in-patient medication required:

Ciprofloxacin 250 mg Tablets X 10

Prescriber: June Littlewood   Bleep: 2134

the ward's nursing staff according to the directions on the inpatient chart, it is not necessary to include administration details on the label.

Labels (we have assumed that the name and address of the pharmacy and the words 'Keep out of the reach and sight of children' are pre-printed on the label) are shown in Figure 11.5.

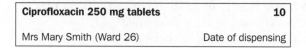

Ciprofloxacin 250 mg tablets	10
Mrs Mary Smith (Ward 26)	Date of dispensing

Figure 11.5

9. **Endorse prescription**
   Endorse the inpatient order with the details of the medication supplied.
10. **Destination of paperwork**
    File the inpatient order within the hospital according to local procedures.
11. **Identity check/counselling**
    Not necessary as the medication will be administered by the nursing staff to the patient on the ward.

Question 2

1. **Identity of order**
   Outpatient prescription.
2. **Prescriber**
   Doctor (hospital consultant).
3. **Legally written?**
   Yes.

4. **Clinical check (complete Table 11.6).**

Table 11.6

Drug	Indications	Dose check	Reference
Ketorolac	Short-term management of moderate-to-severe acute postoperative pain only	Adult and child over 16 years, by mouth, 10 mg every 4–6 h (elderly every 6–8 h) as required; max. 40 mg daily; max. duration of treatment 7 days	*British National Formulary*, 56th edn, section 15.1.4.2

5. **Interactions**
    There is only one item on the prescription form. However, it would also be advisable for the pharmacist or pharmacy technician to check, where possible, the PMR for any concurrent medication that could cause an interaction.

6. **Suitability for patient**
    The item prescribed is safe and suitable for an adult patient and the dose ordered on the prescription is within the recommended dose limits.

7. **Records to be made (including copies of the record[s])**
    None.

8. **Process prescription (including example of label[s])**
    -   Prepare label for product.
    -   Check appendix 9 of the *British National Formulary* for supplementary labelling requirements
        Ketorolac: *British National Formulary* label numbers 17 (Do not take more than . . . in 24 hours) and 21 (. . . with or after food).
    -   Select ketorolac from shelf, remembering to check the expiry date.
    -   Perform final check of item, label and prescription.
    -   Pack in a suitable bag ready to give to patient/patient's representative.
    Labels (we have assumed that the name and address of the pharmacy and the words 'Keep out of the reach and sight of children' are pre-printed on the label.) (Figure 11.6).

Figure 11.6

Ketorolac 10 mg Tablets	20
Take ONE every four to six hours with or after food as directed. Do not take more than 4 in 24 hours.	
Mr Anthony Greenwood	Date of dispensing

9. **Endorse prescription**
    Endorse the outpatient prescription with the details of the medication supplied and initials of the pharmacist and pharmacy technician(s) involved in the dispensing process.

10. **Destination of paperwork**
    File the prescription within the hospital according to local procedures.

11. **Identity check/counselling**
    -   Check patient's name and address.

- Reinforce dosage instructions and that the patient should not take more than four tablets in a 24-hour period.
- Draw patient's attention to the PIL and ask if he has any questions.

Question 3

1. **Identity of order**
   Hospital TTO (TTA) discharge prescription.
2. **Prescriber**
   Doctor (hospital doctor).
3. **Legally written?**
   Yes.
4. **Clinical check (complete Table 11.7).**

Table 11.7

Drug	Indications	Dose check	Reference
Amlodipine	Hypertension, prophylaxis of angina	Initially 5 mg once daily; max. 10 mg once daily	*British National Formulary*, 56th edn, section 2.6.2

5. **Interactions**
   There is only one drug on the TTO. However, it would also be advisable for the pharmacist or pharmacy technician to check the patient's inpatient chart for any concurrent medication that could cause an interaction. Although a patient would need to continue to take all prescribed medication upon discharge, he or she may already have enough of some medication so that medication may not appear on the TTO. This situation is especially likely to occur if the patient is part of a patients' own drugs (POD) scheme.
6. **Suitability for patient**
   Item prescribed is safe and suitable for a patient of this age and the dose ordered on the prescription is within the recommended dose limits.
7. **Records to be made (including copies of the record[s])**
   None.
8. **Process prescription (including example of label[s])**
   - The quantity of medication to be supplied has not been stated. For most medication, the quantity supplied would be based on hospital policy (usually around 14 days). For 14 days' supply, you would need to supply 14 dosage units.
   - Check appendix 9 of the *British National Formulary* for supplementary labelling requirements (there are none).
   - Select amlodipine tablets from shelf, remembering to check expiry date.
   - Perform final check of item, label and prescription.
   - Pack in a suitable bag ready to give to patient/patient's representative.
   Labels (we have assumed that the name and address of the pharmacy and the words 'Keep out of the reach and sight of children' are pre-printed on the label) (Figure 11.7).

Figure 11.7

Amlodipine 10 mg Tablets	14
Take ONE tablet every day.	
Mr Bob Cooper	Date of dispensing

9. **Endorse prescription**
   Endorse the pharmacy box on the TTO with the details of the medication supplied and initials of the pharmacist and pharmacy technician(s) involved in the dispensing process.
10. **Destination of paperwork**
    Either the original or a copy of the TTO is kept with the patient's hospital notes at the hospital. In addition, a copy may be supplied to the patient's GP.
11. **Identity check/counselling**
    The medication must be given to the patient. In most cases, either the patient comes down to the pharmacy to collect the medication as he or she leaves the hospital or the medication is sent to the patient's ward and given to him or her by the ward pharmacist or a member of the nursing staff upon discharge. In both cases, the following information needs to be given to the patient or his representative.
    - Check patient's name and address.
    - Reinforce dosage instructions.
    - Draw patient's attention to the PIL and ask if he has any questions.

Chapter 5

Question 1
1. **Identity of order**
   Private prescription.
2. **Prescriber**
   Dentist (the prescriber is a local dentist).
3. **Legally written?**
   Yes. The item (carbamazepine tablets) is not listed within the *Dental Practitioners' Formulary*; however, as this is a private prescription form, the dentist is not limited to prescribing from within this list.
   Nevertheless, you should still ensure that the dentist is prescribing within his or her area of competence. Carbamazepine is commonly used to treat epilepsy (not something that would usually be within a dentist's area of competence). However, it is also used (among other indications) for the treatment of trigeminal neuralgia, something that would be suitable for treatment by a dentist.

4. Clinical check (complete Table 11.8).

Table 11.8

Drug	Indications	Dose check	Reference
Carbamazepine	Trigeminal neuralgia	Initially 100 mg once or twice daily; usual dose 200 mg three to four times daily; up to 1.6 g daily in some patients	*British National Formulary*, 56th edn, section 2.4

5. **Interactions**

There is only one item on the prescription form. However, it would also be advisable for the pharmacist or pharmacy technician to check the PMR for any concurrent medication that could cause an interaction.

6. **Suitability for patient**

The item prescribed is safe and suitable for an adult patient and the dose ordered on the prescription is within the recommended dose limits.

7. **Records to be made (including copies of the record[s])**

A prescription-only medicines (POM) register entry will be required (Figure 11.8).

Figure 11.8

Reference number	Details	Cost
5.03

Date of supply | Mr Jonathan Jones

135 Knight Street

Anytown

Carbamazepine 100 mg tablets

1 bd

Mitte 28

W. Drillett BDS

Anytown Dental Surgery

Anytown

AN1 1RB

Date on prescription: Today's | Cost
+
50%
+
Dispensing fee
+
Container fee |

8. **Process prescription (including example of label[s])**
    - Prepare product label.
    - Check appendix 9 of the *British National Formulary* for supplementary labelling requirements:

        Carbamazepine: *British National Formulary* label number 3 (Warning: may cause drowsiness. If affected do not drive or operate machinery). As the carbamazepine is being prescribed by a dentist for the treatment of trigeminal neuralgia, label 8 (Do not stop taking this medicine except on your doctor's advice) is not applicable.

- Select carbamazepine tablets from shelf, remembering to check expiry date.
- Perform final check of item, label and prescription.
- Pack in a suitable bag ready to give to patient/patient's representative.

Labels (we have assumed that the name and address of the pharmacy and the words 'Keep out of the reach and sight of children' are pre-printed on the label) (Figure 11.9).

Figure 11.9

Carbamezepine 100 mg Tablets	28
Take ONE tablet twice a day.	
Warning. May cause drowsiness. If affected	
do not drive or operate machinery.	
Mr Jonathan Jones	Date of dispensing

9. **Endorse prescription**
   Stamp with pharmacy stamp to indicate completion and annotate stamp with the POM register entry number (5.03).
10. **Destination of paperwork**
    Retain prescription in pharmacy for 2 years.
11. **Identity check/counselling**
    - Check patient's name and address.
    - Reinforce the dosage instructions.
    - Advise the patient that the tablets may cause drowsiness and, if affected, not to drive or operate machinery.
    - If the patient has not had the medication before, you need to advise him about potential blood, hepatic or skin disorders (see *British National Formulary*, section 4.8.1, for details).
    - Draw patient's attention to the PIL and ask if he has any questions.

Question 2

1. **Identity of order**
   Private prescription.
2. **Prescriber**
   Doctor (the prescriber is a local doctor).
3. **Legally written?**
   Yes.
4. **Clinical check (complete Table 11.9).**

Table 11.9

Drug	Indications	Dose check	Reference
Atenolol	Angina	100 mg daily in 1 or 2 doses	*British National Formulary*, 56th edn, section 4.8.1

5. **Interactions**
   There is only one item on the prescription form. However, it would also be advisable for the pharmacist or pharmacy technician to check the PMR for any concurrent medication that could cause an interaction.

6. **Suitability for patient**

   The item prescribed is safe and suitable for an adult patient and the dose ordered on the prescription is within the recommended dose limits.

7. **Records to be made (including copies of the record[s])**

   A POM register entry will be required (Figure 11.10).

Figure 11.10

Reference number	Details	Cost
5.04 Date of supply	Mrs Emma Taylor 6 Windmill Close Anytown Atenolol 100 mg tablets 1 od Mitte 28 R U Better MB ChB Anytown Health Centre Anytown, AN1 1RB Date on prescription: Today's	Cost + 50% + Dispensing fee + Container fee

8. **Process prescription (including example of label[s])**

   ■ Prepare product label.

   ■ Check appendix 9 of the *British National Formulary* for supplementary labelling requirements:

   > Atenolol: *British National Formulary* label number 8 (Do not stop taking this medicine except on your doctor's advice.).

   ■ Select atenolol tablets from shelf, remembering to check expiry date.

   ■ Perform final check of item, label and prescription.

   ■ Pack in a suitable bag ready to give to patient/patient's representative.

   Labels (we have assumed that the name and address of the pharmacy and the words 'Keep out of the reach and sight of children' are pre-printed on the label.) (Figure 11.11).

Athenolol 100 mg Tablets	28
Take ONE tablet daily. Do not stop taking this medicine except on your doctor's advice.	
Mrs Emma Taylor	Date of dispensing

Figure 11.11

9. **Endorse prescription**

   Stamp with pharmacy stamp to indicate completion and annotate stamp with the POM register entry number (5.04).

10. **Destination of paperwork**
    Retain prescription in pharmacy for 2 years.
11. **Identity check/counselling**
    - Check patient's name and address.
    - Reinforce the dosage instructions and that the patient should not stop taking the medication without seeking advice.
    - Draw patient's attention to the PIL and ask if she has any questions.

Question 3

1. **Identity of order**
   Written requisition.
2. **Requisitioner**
   Dentist (the requisitioner is a local dentist).
3. **Legally written?**
   No. The requisition needs to state the purpose of the requisition and the strength of the amoxicillin injections required (250 mg, 500 mg and 1 g vials are available).
4. **Records to be made (including copies of the record[s])**
   A POM register entry will be required (although as the written requisition can be kept for 2 years, the entry is only good practice) (Figure 11.12).

Figure 11.12

Reference number	Details	Cost
5.05 Date of supply	Wilbur Drillett BDS Anytown Dental Surgery Anytown AN1 1RB Please supply: 10 Amoxicillin Injections W Drillett Date on requisition: Today's Dentist contacted for additions of purpose (for use in surgery) and for strength of injections required (250 mg).	Cost + 50% + VAT

5. **Process requisition**
   - Select a full original pack from the shelf to sell to the dentist without labelling.
   - Check expiry date; make final check of item against the requisition.
   - Pack in a suitable bag ready to give to dentist.

6. **Endorse requisition**
   Stamp with pharmacy stamp to indicate completion and annotate stamp with the POM register entry number (5.05).
7. **Destination of paperwork**
   Retain requisition in pharmacy for 2 years.
8. **Identity check/counselling**
   Check identity of person collecting.

Question 4

1. **Identity of order**
   Written requisition.
2. **Requisitioner**
   Optometrist.
3. **Legally written?**
   No. The requisition needs to indicate that the individual is an optometrist (usually by the inclusion of the optician's qualifications) and state the purpose of the requisition. In addition, pilocarpine can be supplied only to an additional supply optometrist (see *Applied Pharmaceutical Practice* (Langley and Belcher, 2008)) so this would also need to be confirmed before the supply can be made.
4. **Records to be made (including copies of the record[s])**
   A POM register entry will be required (although as the written requisition can be kept for 2 years, the entry is only good practice) (Figure 11.13).

Figure 11.13

Reference number	Details	Cost
5.06 Date of supply	Miss C Ittall Anytown Opticians High Street, ANYTOWN AN1 1RB Please supply: Pilocarpine Hydrochloride 1% eye drops 1 X OP C Ittall Date on requisition: Today's Optician contacted for addition of qualification (MBCO) and confirmation that she is an additional supply optometrist. Also contacted for the purpose (for use in practice.).	Cost + 50% + VAT

5. **Process requisition**
   - Select a full original pack from the shelf to sell to the optometrist without labelling.
   - Check expiry date; make final check of item against the requisition.
   - Pack in a suitable bag ready to give to optometrist.
6. **Endorse requisition**
   Stamp with pharmacy stamp to indicate completion and annotate stamp with the POM register entry number (5.06).
7. **Destination of paperwork**
   Retain requisition in pharmacy for 2 years.
8. **Identity check/counselling**
   Check identity of person collecting.

Chapter 6

Question 1
Answer: A
Schedule 1
Controlled drugs in Schedule 1 cannot be routinely prescribed.

Question 2
Answer: D
Specify the total quality of drug in both words and figures.
The total quantity needs to be stated but this does not need to be in both words and figures.

Question 3
Answer: C
Statement (1) is correct but statement (2) is incorrect.
The supply of a Schedule 3 controlled drug on a requisition does not need to be recorded legally in the POM register but this is because a photocopy of the requisition will be kept at the premises (as the original will be sent to the PPD [or equivalent] for monitoring purposes). The supply of Schedule 3 controlled drugs would not be recorded in the controlled drugs register.

Question 4
Answer: B
A specific start date must be stated.
Instalment prescriptions may specify a start date but they do not have to.

Question 5
1. **Identity of order**
   NHS prescription (FP10SS). The prescription is for a drug that is classified as a Schedule 2 controlled drug, so the additional requirements relating to Schedule 2 controlled drugs need to be met before the prescription can be dispensed.

2. **Prescriber**
   Doctor (GP).

3. **Legally written?**
   No. As the prescription is for a Schedule 2 controlled drug, additional prescription requirements need to be met before the prescription can be dispensed. In this case, the dose to be taken is missing from the prescription form and, in addition, without details of the frequency of administration, it is not possible to verify whether the prescriber has limited the supply to 30 days (a good practice requirement). The usual dose frequency for modified-release methylphenidate (i.e. Concerta XL in this case) is once daily (suggesting that this would be 120 days' supply).

4. **Clinical check (complete Table 11.10).**

Table 11.10

Drug	Indications	Dose check	Reference
Methylphenidate (Concerta XL)	Attention deficit hyperactivity disorder	Modified release: child over 6 years, initially 18 mg once daily (in the morning), increased if necessary in weekly steps of 18 mg according to response; max. 54 mg once daily	*British National Formulary*, 56th edn, section 4.4

5. **Interactions**
   There is only one drug on the prescription. However, it would also be advisable for the pharmacist or pharmacy technician to check the PMR for any concurrent medication that could cause an interaction.

6. **Suitability for patient**
   As detailed above, there is no indication of the frequency of administration. This needs to be added to the prescription by the prescriber before it can legally be supplied (suggest one tablet to be taken in the morning). In addition, it would be sensible to speak to the prescriber and establish whether there is a need to prescribe more than 30 days' supply.

7. **Item(s) allowable on the NHS**
   Yes (see *Drug Tariff*).

8. **Records to be made (including copies of the record[s])**
   An entry would need to be made to the relevant section of the controlled drugs register detailing the supply. In addition a note of the intervention (regarding the missed dosage instructions and the number of days' supply) on a clinical intervention form would be made (Figure 11.14).

9. **Process prescription (including example of label[s])**
   - Prepare label for product.
   - Check appendix 9 of *British National Formulary* for supplementary labelling requirements.
       Methylphenidate: *British National Formulary* label number 25 (. . . swallowed whole, not chewed).
   - Select pack of methylphenidate (Concerta XL) from the controlled drugs cupboard, remembering to check the expiry date.
   - Perform final check of item, label and prescription.

Figure 11.14

MISUSE OF DRUGS ACT
REGISTER OF:

DRUG CLASS *Methylphenidate*

NAME (brand, strength, form) *ConcertaXL36 mg tablets*

Date	Obtained		Supplied							Balance
supply received or date supplied	Name, address of person or firm from whom obtained	Amount Obtained	Name, address of person or firm supplied	Authority to possess-presciber or licence holder details	Person collecting Patient/Representative or Healthcare Professional (name and address)	Proof of identity requested Yes/No	Proof of identity provided Yes/No	Amount supplied		Carried over: 200
Today's			*Sharon Carr* *32 Holly Hill* *Anytown*	*Dr R U Better* *FP10*	*Representative* *(mother)*	*Yes*	*Yes*	*120*		*80*

- Pack in a suitable bag ready to give to the patient or patient's representative (as this is a Schedule 2 controlled drug, it should be kept in the controlled drugs cupboard until it is collected by the patient or representative).

Labels (we have assumed that the name and address of the pharmacy and the words 'Keep out of the reach and sight of children' are pre-printed on the label) (Figure 11.15).

Figure 11.15

Methylphenidate 36 mg m/r Tablets	**120**
Take ONE tablet every morning swallowed whole, not chewed.	
Miss Sharon Carr	Date of dispensing

10. **Endorse prescription**
   Stamp with pharmacy stamp to indicate completion and mark the date of supply.
11. **Destination of paperwork**
   Send to the PPD at the end of the month. The controlled drugs register in which the details of the supply were made must be kept at the premises at all times during use and for 2 years from the last date of entry.
12. **Identity check/counselling**
   - Check patient's name and address.
   - The pharmacist or pharmacy technician must identify whether the collector is the patient, patient's representative or a healthcare professional. This information (including the name and professional address if the collector is a healthcare professional) must be recorded in the controlled drugs register.
   - The pharmacist or pharmacy technician must note in the controlled drugs register whether ID was requested from the collector and whether it was produced.

- The collector should be asked to sign the rear of the prescription form.
- Reinforce the dosage instructions; advise that the tablets are to be swallowed whole and not chewed.
- Draw patient's representative's attention to the PIL and ask if she has any questions.

Question 6

1. **Identity of order**

   Private prescription. The prescription is for a drug that is classified as a Schedule 3 controlled drug, so the additional requirements relating to Schedule 3 controlled drugs need to be met before the prescription can be dispensed.

2. **Prescriber**

   Doctor (general practitioner).

3. **Legally written?**

   No. The doctor has failed to add the patient's address to the prescription and (although we may know from local knowledge) there is also no indication of type of prescriber on the prescription. This is usually indicated by the addition of qualifications to the prescription. In addition, as the prescription is on a private (non-NHS) prescription form for a Schedule 3 controlled drug for dispensing within the community (for human use), the prescription needs to be on an FP10PCD and contain the prescriber's private prescriber indentification number.

4. **Clinical check (complete Table 11.11)**

Table 11.11

Drug	Indications	Dose check	Reference
Phenobarbital	All forms of epilepsy except absence seizures; status epilepticus	By mouth, 60–180 mg at night	*British National Formulary*, 56th edn, section 4.8.2

5. **Interactions**

   There is only one drug on the prescription form. However, it would also be advisable for the pharmacist or pharmacy technician to check the PMR for any concurrent medication that could cause an interaction.

6. **Suitability for patient**

   The item prescribed is safe and suitable for an adult patient and the dose ordered on the prescription is within the recommended dose limits.

7. **Item(s) allowable on the NHS**

   N/A (this is a private [non-NHS] prescription).

8. **Records to be made (including copies of the record[s])**

   As the supply is for a Schedule 3 controlled drug, the pharmacist does not need to make an entry in the controlled drugs register detailing the supply. However, it is necessary to make an entry within the POM register (including details of the intervention) (Figure 11.16).

Figure 11.16

Reference number	Details	Cost
6.01 Date of supply	Mrs Sheila Smith 15 Boot Lane, Anytown Phenobarbital 30 mg tablets 2 to be taken at night Mitte 56 (fifty-six) R U Better MB ChB (Private Prescriber Identification Number: 666666) Anytown Health Centre Anytown R U Better MB ChB Date on requisition: Today's Prescriber contacted to transfer prescription to an FP10PCD (original prescription not on an FP10PCD and omitted patient's address and prescriber's qualifications).	Cost + 50% + Dispensing fee + Container fee

9. **Process prescription (including example of label(s)**
   - Prepare label for product.
   - Check appendix 9 of *British National Formulary* for supplementary labelling requirements:
     Phenobarbital: *British National Formulary* label numbers 2 (Warning: may cause drowsiness. If affected do not drive or operate machinery. Avoid alcoholic drink) and 8 (Do not stop taking this medicine except on your doctor's advice.).
   - Select pack of phenobarbital from the shelf, remembering to check the expiry date.
   - Perform final check of item, label and prescription.
   - Pack in a suitable bag ready to give to the patient or patient's representative.
   Labels (we have assumed that the name and address of the pharmacy and the words 'Keep out of the reach and sight of children' are pre-printed on the label) (Figure 11.17).

Figure 11.17

Phenobarbital 30 mg Tablets	**56**
Take TWO tablets every night. Warning. May cause drowsiness. If affected do not drive or operate machinery. Avoid alcoholic drink. Do not stop taking this medicine except on your doctor's advice.	
Mrs Sheila Smith	Date of dispensing

10. **Endorse prescription**

   Stamp with pharmacy stamp to indicate completion and annotate stamp with the POM register entry number (6.01).

11. **Destination of paperwork**

   Send to the PPD at the end of the month. It would be good practice to keep a photocopy of the prescription for your records.

12. **Identity check/counselling**

   - Check patient's name and address.
   - The collector should be asked to sign the rear of the prescription form.
   - If the patient has not had the medication before, you need to advise her about driving while taking the medication (see *British National Formulary*, section 4.8.1 for details).
   - Reinforce the dosage instructions; advise that the patient should take two tablets at night and not to stop taking the medication unless advised.
   - Inform the patient that the tablets may make her feel drowsy and, if she is affected, she should not drive or operate machinery; this effect is likely to be enhanced by alcohol.
   - Draw the patient's attention to the PIL and ask if she has any questions.

Question 7

1. **Identity of order**

   NHS prescription (FP10SS). The prescription is for a drug that is classified as a Schedule 2 controlled drug, so the additional requirements relating to Schedule 2 controlled drugs need to be met before the prescription can be dispensed.

2. **Prescriber**

   Doctor (GP).

3. **Legally written?**

   Yes. As the prescription is for a Schedule 2 controlled drug, additional prescription requirements need to be met before the prescription can be dispensed. In this case, all the additional legal requirements for a prescription for a Schedule 2 controlled drug have been met.

4. **Clinical check (complete Table 11.12).**

Table 11.12

Drug	Indications	Dose check	Reference
Morphine (MST)	Acute pain	10 mg every 12 h adjusted according to response	*British National Formulary*, 56th edn, section 4.7.2

5. **Interactions**

   There is only one drug on the prescription. However, it would also be advisable for the pharmacist or pharmacy technician to check the PMR for any concurrent medication that could cause an interaction.

6. **Suitability for patient**

   Although all the prescription requirements for a Schedule 2 controlled drug have been met, the prescriber has prescribed the item four times a day. MST tablets are a sustained-release form of morphine and are usually prescribed twice a day. The dosage will need to be queried with the prescriber before the item is dispensed.

7. **Item(s) allowable on the NHS**
   Yes (see *Drug Tariff*).

8. **Records to be made (including copies of the record[s])**
   An entry would need to be made in the relevant section of the controlled drugs register detailing the supply. In addition a note of the intervention would be made on a clinical intervention form.

Figure 11.18

Date	Obtained			Supplied							Balance
supply received or date supplied	Name, address of person or firm from whom obtained	Amount Obtained		Name, address of person or firm supplied	Authority to possess-prescriber or licence holder details	Person collecting		Proof of identity requested Yes/No	Proof of identity provided Yes/No	Amount supplied	Carried over:
						Patient/Representative or Healthcare Professional (name and address)					120
Today's				Samantha Brown 134 High Street Anytown	Dr R U Better FP10	Patient		Yes	Yes	60	60

9. **Process prescription (including example of label[s])**
   - Prepare label for product
   - Check appendix 9 of British *National Formulary* for supplementary labelling requirements:
     MST: *British National Formulary* label numbers 2 (Warning: may cause drowsiness. If affected do not drive or operate machinery. Avoid alcoholic drink) and 25 (. . . swallowed whole, not chewed).
   - Select pack of MST from the controlled drugs cupboard, remembering to check the expiry date and taking care that the correct strength of drug has been selected (the packaging of other strengths is very similar).
   - Perform final check of item, label and prescription.
   - Pack in a suitable bag ready to give to the patient or patient's representative (as this is a Schedule 2 controlled drug, it should be kept in the controlled drugs cupboard until it is collected by the patient or her representative).

   Labels (we have assumed that the name and address of the pharmacy and the words 'Keep out of the reach and sight of children' are pre-printed on the label) (Figure 11.19).

Figure 11.19

MST Continus 10 mg Tablets	60
Take ONE tablet twice a day swallowed whole not chewed. Warning. May cause drowsiness. If affected do not drive or operate machinery. Avoid alcoholic drink.	
Mrs Sheila Smith	Date of dispensing

10. Endorse prescription

Stamp with pharmacy stamp to indicate completion and mark the date of supply.

11. Destination of paperwork

Send to the PPD at the end of the month. The controlled drugs register in which the details of the supply were made must be kept at the premises at all times during use and for 2 years from the last date of entry.

12. Identity check/counselling

- Check patient's name and address.
- The pharmacist or pharmacy technician must identify whether the collector is the patient, patient's representative or a healthcare professional. This information (including the name and professional address if the collector is a healthcare professional) must be recorded in the controlled drugs register.
- The pharmacist or pharmacy technician must note in the controlled drugs register whether ID was requested from the collector and whether it was produced.
- The collector should be asked to sign the rear of the prescription form.
- Reinforce the dosage instructions; advise that the tablets are best taken 12 hours apart, with or after food, and may cause drowsiness.
- Draw patient's attention to the PIL and ask if she has any questions.

Chapter 7

Question 1

Answer: C

Date on which the prescription is received.

The age of the patient is legally required only if the patient is under 12 years of age. The dose of the medication does not legally have to be supplied because 'as directed' would be legally acceptable. There is no legal requirement to annotate the POM register with any specific words regarding emergency supply. The doctor's qualifications are not legally required; most patients could tell you who their GP is and most could supply an address but very few if any would know their GP's qualifications.

Question 2

Answer: B

Buprenorphine 200 microgram tablets.

Buprenorphine is a Schedule 3 controlled drug and cannot be supplied under the emergency supply regulations.

Question 3
Answer: E
The words 'Emergency supply'.
When an item is requested to be supplied as an emergency by a prescriber, the labelling requirements are exactly the same as those for the supply of any medicine on a prescription.

Question 4
Answer: A
Veterinary surgeon.
All others may request emergency supplies.

Question 5
Answer: D
The first statement is false but the second statement is true.
In this situation the phenobarbital could be supplied under the emergency supply regulations because it is for use in the treatment of epilepsy.

Question 6
Answer: D
The first statement is false but the second statement is true. Dentists are allowed to request items using the emergency supply regulations.
Statement 2 is true but has no bearing on the issue of supply.

Question 7
Answer: A
Both statements are true and the second statement is a correct explanation of the first statement.
To legally supply a pharmacist should interview the patient NOT the representative, so under the circumstances outlined it would not be legally correct to supply and the reason is that it is her representative who is requesting the medication.

Question 8
Answer: E
Statement 3 is correct and statements 1 and 2 are incorrect.
There is no requirement to contact a patient's GP before supplying and only medicines supplied as an emergency supply at the request of a patient need to be labelled 'Emergency supply'. Remember, emergency supplies of controlled drugs at the request of a patient (i.e. phenobarbital or phenobarbital sodium for the treatement of epilepsy or any Schedule 4 or 5 controlled drug) are limited to a maximum of 5 days' treatment.

Question 9
Answer: B
Statements 1 and 2 are correct and statement 3 is incorrect.
There is no provision in the regulations to allow patients to obtain subsequent emergency supplies without visiting their GP.

Question 10
Answer: D
Statement 1 is correct and statements 2 and 3 are incorrect.
The pharmacist is allowed to provide a complete cycle in the case of emergency supply of contraceptives and an emergency supply to a patient does not involve the promise to supply a prescription.

Chapter 8

Question 1
Answer: C
O stands for 'Other symptoms'.
O actually stands for 'Observe'.

Question 2
Answer: D
H stands for 'History of medicines taken'.
H actually stands for 'History of any disease or condition'.

Question 3
Answer: B
W stands for 'What medicines have been tried?'.
The second W actually stands for 'What are the symptoms?'.

Question 4
Answer: C
D stands for 'Doing anything to alleviate the condition'.
D actually stands for 'Duration'.

Question 5
Answer: A
What is your name?
B is an open question, C is a probing question and D is a prompting question.

Question 6
Answer: B
Open questions.
Open questions give the opportunity for patients to provide all the information themselves.

Question 7
Answer: B
Avoid eye contact.

Question 8
Answer: A
Fever.
Slurred speech could indicate a lesion in the brain (tumour or abscess). Neck stiffness is one of the symptoms of meningitis, a life-threatening condition, and drowsiness, visual disturbances and vomiting could indicate a haemorrhage that could have been caused by trauma.

Question 9
Answer: D
Non-productive, dry, tickly cough associated with a cold.
Such coughs are usually viral in nature and self-limiting. Chest pain is always referred; the lung tissue feels no pain and pain can suggest pleurisy or pulmonary embolism. Children suffering regular night-time cough without associated cold symptoms may be showing signs of asthma and therefore need referral. Blood in sputum could suggest tuberculosis or cancer and also need urgent referral.

Question 10
Answer: A
Vaginal discharge.
Abdominal pain may suggest that the irritation is caused by a urinary infection that may need medical attention. Vaginal infections in people with diabetes can indicate poor diabetic control resulting in sugar in the urine. Vaginal infections when pregnant are always referred on.

Question 11
Answer: C
Lactulose.
Stimulant laxatives can result in an anatomical non-functioning colon and liquid paraffin is no longer recommended for long-term use. Lactulose is the drug of choice

Question 12
Answer: D
Statement 1 is correct and statements 2 and 3 are incorrect.
Quite often there is no itching associated with head lice (which develops as an allergic response to the saliva of the lice). Lice have no preference with regard to the cleanliness of hair, its colour or its length.

Question 13
Answer: B
Statements 1 and 2 are correct and statement 3 is incorrect.
Routine use of head lice treatments is not recommended because this can lead
to resistance developing to the insecticides used.

Question 14
Answer: B
Statements 1 and 2 are correct and statement 3 is incorrect.
Cradle cap is not contagious but is common in infants.

Question 15
Answer: B
Statements 1 and 2 are correct and statement 3 is incorrect.
Before treating any foot complaint it is important to check whether the patient
has diabetes because this may affect the peripheral circulation and therefore the
ability to heal. The symptoms suggest that the patient has a verruca so salicylic
acid would be an appropriate recommendation for treatment. Referral to a
doctor would be inappropriate because warts and verrucas may spontaneously
disappear and in general are not a risk to health in an otherwise healthy adult.

Question 16
Answer: C
Statements 2 and 3 are correct and statement 1 is incorrect.
Chickenpox is caused by varicella-zoster virus. People with active shingles are
contagious to people who have never had chickenpox. The reverse is not true;
shingles cannot be caught from a person suffering from chickenpox and is an
'old wives' tale'. Promethazine is an antihistamine that helps prevent itching
and also has the side effect of causing drowsiness, which means that when
itching is a problem a night-time dose may aid sleep.

Question 17
Answer: A
Statements 1, 2 and 3 are all correct.
All are symptoms of tinea pedis.

Question 18
Answer: C
Statements 2 and 3 are correct and statement 1 is incorrect.
Sitting on radiator, etc., may be uncomfortable but will not cause haemorrhoids;
this is a popular 'old wives' tale'.

Question 19
Answer: B
Statements 1 and 2 are correct and statement 3 is incorrect.
It is important for the patient to realise that this is a potent cream which should
not be applied liberally as with an emollient; details as to what is meant by a

fingertip unit may need to be expanded upon. An occlusive dressing, such as a plastic glove, is not recommended because this can increase systemic absorption.

Question 20
Answer: B
Statements 1 and 2 are correct and statement 3 is incorrect.
Lactulose is an osmotic laxative and Fybogel a bulk-forming laxative so they exert their action in different ways.

Chapter 9

Question 1
- Wash hands.
- Wash area (preferably with an emollient wash) and pat dry gently with a towel (do not rub).
- Apply the cream or ointment sparingly (thinly) to the affected area.
- Gently massage the cream or ointment into the skin.
- After application wash hands again unless the hands are the area being treated.
- Use two fingertip units at each application.
- A fingertip unit is the amount of cream that can be placed from the tip to the first crease of an adult index finger.
- You should leave 30 minutes between the application of the emollient and application of the steroid cream. There is no consensus as to the order in which the creams should be applied. The order should be guided by patient preference and any routine that ensures compliance should be encouraged. The time between the applications (i.e. 30 minutes) is the important factor.
- A soap substitute that could be recommended is to actually use the aqueous cream as a soap substitute. Alternatively, emulsifying ointment or other proprietary products could be recommended.
- The application of Clingfilm to the feet would act as an occlusive dressing and this is not recommended with steroid creams because it encourages more systemic absorption of the drug.

Question 2
- Take three 5 mL spoonfuls of the solution twice a day. Measure using the 5 mL spoon provided. Take the medication regularly.
- It can take up to 3 days to work.
- It may cause bloating and an increase in flatulence (wind) for the first few days of treatment, but this usually clears if the treatment is continued.
- If you find lactulose unpleasant to take, it may be mixed with water, fruit juice or squash.
- Whether or not you will need to keep taking laxatives depends on the cause of the constipation. Constipation can be a symptom of an underlying condition for which the doctor will test if you need to keep taking the medication. Alternatively, are you taking any other medication because constipation can be a side effect of some medications?

- Constipation is a common condition but there are steps that you can take to help prevent it or alleviate the condition. Ensure that you have sufficient fibre in your diet by eating more fruit, vegetables, nuts, seeds, oats, and wholemeal varieties of pasta and bread (increase fibre intake gradually to prevent stomach cramps caused by excess wind). The fibre helps to keep the contents of the bowel moving and helps other food to pass through, thus reducing the chance of constipation. Increase in fluid intake will also help as will increased exercise.
- You should also never ignore the urge to pass stools because this can considerably increase the chances of constipation.
- Lactulose does not work in the same way as Fybogel. Lactulose works by softening the stools through an increase in the amount of water retained in the bowel, whereas Fybogel is a bulk-forming laxative and works by increasing the volume of the content of the bowel; this stimulates the bowel muscle to push the contents along the bowel more quickly and prevent constipation. Fybogel is normally used only when increases in dietary fibre have failed.

Question 3

- Wash hands with soapy water before using eyedrops.
- If necessary clean the eyes with boiled and cooled water and a tissue (one tissue for each eye) to remove any discharge or remaining wateriness (do not use cotton wool because it may leave fibres behind that may irritate the eye).
- Shake the bottle of drops if necessary. Some eyedrops are suspensions and will need shaking; if applicable, this direction will be on the label.
- Remove the lid from the bottle.
- Relax and either sit down or lie down and tilt the head backwards so that you are looking at the ceiling.
- Gently pull down the lower eyelid with a finger to make a pocket between the eye and the lower eyelid.
- Look upwards.
- Rest the dropper bottle on the forehead above the eye.
- Squeeze one drop inside the lower eyelid (do not allow the dropper tip to touch the eye).
- Close the eye and gently blot away any excess drops on a clean tissue.
- Apply slight pressure to the inner corner of the eye for about 30 seconds. This will prevent the drops running down the tear duct and into the back of the throat, avoiding any unpleasant after taste and also minimising any absorption into the body, so minimising possible side effects.
- Replace the lid on the bottle.
- Remember to discard any remaining drops 4 weeks after opening.

As the drops are for use in treatment of glaucoma additional helpful advice may include:

- These drops are to treat glaucoma, which is a permanent condition that will require long-term treatment. To prevent it from getting worse and so preserve your vision it is important that the drops are used regularly.

Sometimes these drops can cause stinging; when administered this can be minimised by storing the drops in the fridge. The cool drops sometimes feel more soothing and, in addition, if you are unsure of your technique when instilling the drops the drops' coolness makes it easier to tell that they have entered the eye. There can be some side effects that affect the body rather than the localised stinging; this can be minimised by applying slight pressure to the inner corner of the eye or alternatively by closing the eyes for 2–3 minutes after instilling the drops. As these drops are for long-term therapy it may be helpful to store your drops near your toothbrush, for example, so that you remember to use the drops twice a day.

- If the stinging persists and is a problem, see your ophthalmologist because it could be the preservative in the medication that is causing the problem. Should you notice any breathlessness when using these drops, stop using them and return to your GP.
- Glaucoma is not catching. It is not caused by diet or lifestyle. At present it is not preventable and seems to be part of the natural ageing process of some individuals. Regular eye checks will ensure that the condition is detected early and can therefore be treated early. Sight tests are free to patients with glaucoma and also their brothers, sisters and children. Therefore regular visits to the optometrist will ensure that the condition is detected. They may never develop glaucoma.
- Legally you must inform the DVLA and your insurance company of any significant change in sight that may affect the safety of your driving, e.g. if both eyes are affected by glaucoma. They may request that you visit an optometrist registered with them for an appropriate field of vision test. Patients with glaucoma rarely go blind, provided that they use the medication as prescribed and attend regular check-ups.

Question 4

- Mrs Jones, the Gaviscon Advance liquid supplied by your doctor should be taken three times a day after food and at bedtime. You need to take two 5 mL spoonfuls at each dose using the spoon provided. Ideally the medicine should be taken while standing or at least sitting upright.
- Pick up the container with the label against the palm of the hand, to protect the label from staining by any dripping medicine.
- Shake the bottle and measure the dose on to the spoon.
- Transfer to the mouth and swallow. Once the dose has been taken, clean the neck of the bottle to help prevent the lid sticking, then replace the lid. It is often easier to take the medicine while standing near to a wash basin or sink, making it possible to measure the dose and clean away any accidental spillages with ease.
- Mr Jones should take his oxytetracycline one tablet four times a day on an empty stomach. Swallow whole (not crushed or chewed) with the aid of a glass of water. (Plenty of water ensures that the tablet or capsule reaches the stomach and does not feel like it is 'stuck' in the throat.) It is important to avoid dairy products, such as milk, at the time of taking the tablets because these will stop the oxytetracycline being absorbed.

- The tablets should be taken at regular intervals during waking hours to ensure that the levels of oxytetracycline in the body remain constant; he should complete the course unless otherwise directed by his doctor. This is important even if he feels better because the infection could return and be more difficult to treat.
- It is also important that he does not take indigestion mixtures at the same time as this medication nor should he take iron or zinc supplements. Ideally the tablets should be taken whilst standing or at least sitting upright.
- The patient should not lie down flat for at least 20 minutes to ensure that the tablet gets to the stomach as quickly as possible. Should he forget to take a dose it would be best for him to take the dose as soon as he remembers, unless it is almost time for the next dose in which case he should leave out the missing dose. Never take two doses at the same time to try to 'catch up'.
- If both items were for the same patient, the advice added would be that, as Gaviscon Advance is an antacid and will impair the absorption of oxytetracycline, spacing of the doses of Gaviscon Advance and oxytetracycline will be critical. It is important that they are not taken at the same time. Take the oxytetracycline before food and the Gaviscon Advance after food leaving a gap of 2–3 hours between the time that the oxytetracycline is taken and the time that the Gaviscon Advance is taken.

Question 5

- First assemble the spacer device as directed by the manufacturer (with or without a facemask).
- Remove the cap from the inhaler and insert the mouthpiece of the inhaler into the opening at the end of the spacer.
- Hold the spacer and inhaler together and shake.
- Ask Emily to breathe out.
- Put the spacer mouthpiece in her mouth and seal with her lips.
- Press the inhaler once and she should breathe in and out four or five times.
- Separate the spacer and inhaler. Replace the inhaler cap and store until next dose.
- As Emily has two inhalers you should be aware that the brown inhaler is a preventer and needs to be taken regularly twice a day, even if the symptoms of asthma may seem to have disappeared. The brown preventer inhaler should completely control the symptoms but occasionally Emily may find that her asthma temporarily worsens, so occasionally she may need to use her blue inhaler, which is a reliever.
- The spacer device with its mask can be alarming to young children. It may help if you allow Emily to play with the spacer to familiarise herself with it and even decorate it with pretty stickers.
- The brown inhaler can lead to thrush in the mouth so it is important that Emily rinses her mouth with a drink after using it; similarly the area of her face covered by the mask should also be cleaned/wiped as well.
- It is important that you do not run out of medication for Emily. You can work out how long the inhaler should last and reorder from the doctor before it runs out. For example, the beclometasone (brown) inhaler contains

200 doses, so as Emily has two puffs a day this should last 100 days; mark on the calendar when you expect to need to reorder a prescription. The blue reliever inhaler is used when required so it is a little more difficult to track its usage; to be sure it is advised that a spare blue inhaler should always be kept in stock.

■ A static charge can build up on the inside of the spacer device and attract particles of the drug which stick to the spacer device. This is easily prevented by washing the device in soapy water and leaving to dry naturally. You should also check that the valve at the end of the spacer opens and closes with each breath. It is recommended that the spacer device be replaced every 12 months.

After you have explained the use of the inhaler to her, Mrs Smith is more confident about its use, but asks you if you think that it is likely that Emily will grow out of asthma.

Some children do grow out of asthma, i.e. they lose their symptoms by the time they are adults; others find that their symptoms become milder. There are no strict rules; it varies from case to case. Controlling the symptoms is important so that Emily does not damage her lungs and when she starts school does not need to miss days because of her wheezing.

Chapter 10

Question 1
Answer: E
Statement 3 is correct and statements 1 and 2 are incorrect.
The Poisons Act 1972 superseded the Pharmacy and Poisons Act 1933. The Medicines Act 1968 is concerned with medicinal poisons only.

Question 2
Answer: E
Statement 3 is correct and statements 1 and 2 are incorrect.
The sale of alcohols is covered by more than one piece of legislation.

Question 3
Answer: D
Statement 1 is correct and statements 2 and 3 are incorrect.
Labelling of non-medicinal poisons is governed by CHIP regulations. The Poisons Act 1972 is not law in Northern Ireland.

Question 4
Answer: E
Statement 3 is correct and statements 1 and 2 are incorrect.
Part II non-medicinal poisons may be sold by listed sellers and pharmacies; non-medicinal poisons are controlled by the Poisons Act 1972. However, any medicinal product comes under the control of the Medicines Act 1968, e.g. sodium fluoride is a POM, P or GSL medicine depending on the strength of the

preparation used for the prophylaxis of dental caries, but when sold as a preservative or non-medicinal poison, it is a Part II, Schedule 4 poison.

Question 5
Answer: C
Statements 2 and 3 are correct and statement 1 is incorrect.
Unlike in the case of written requisitions for medicinal products negating the necessity for a POM register entry, the provision of a signed order for a poison is insufficient record and a poisons register entry must be made.

Question 6
Answer: B
Statements 1 and 2 are correct and statement 3 is incorrect.
The date is not legally required; the Home Office has indicated that this should be added and it is therefore good practice to do so.

Question 7
Answer: B
Statements 1 and 2 are correct and statement 3 is incorrect.
There is no limit stated for the quantity of IDA to supply on an NHS prescription.

Question 8
Answer: A
Statements 1, 2 and 3 are all correct.

Question 9
Answer: D
Statement 1 is correct and statements 2 and 3 are incorrect.
The sale of medicinal products is covered by the legislation written in the Medicines Act 1968. When sold as an insecticide, the Poisons Act 1972 is the legislation that covers the sale of nicotine because in this case nicotine is a non-medicinal poison.

Appendix 1
Commonly encountered qualifications of healthcare professionals

Medical practitioners
Governing body: General Medical Council (GMC)

MB, BM	Bachelor of Medicine
MD, DM	Doctor of Medicine (a medical higher degree)
ChB, BChir, BS	Bachelor of Surgery
MRCP	Member of the Royal College of Physicians
MRCS	Member of the Royal College of Surgeons
FRCP	Fellow of the Royal College of Physicians
FRCS	Fellow of the Royal College of Surgeons

Note: it is common for a first degree in medicine to include both a medical and a surgical qualification e.g. MB ChB.

Dentists
Governing body: British Dental Council

BDS, BChD	Bachelor of Dental Surgery
LDS	Licentiate in Dental Surgery

Veterinary surgeons
Governing body: Council of the Royal College of Veterinary Surgeons

MRCVS	Member of the Royal College of Veterinary Surgeons
FRCVS	Fellow of the Royal College of Veterinary Surgeons

Ophthalmic opticians
Governing body: General Optical Council

MCOptom	Member of the College of Optometrists
FCOptom	Fellow of the College of Optometrists
FBOA	Fellowship Diploma of the British Optical Association
MBCO	Member of the British College of Optometrists
FBCO	Fellow of the British College of Optometrists
DCLP	Diploma in Contact Lens Practice

Nurses
Governing body: Central Council for Nursing, Midwifery and Health Visiting

RGN	Registered General Nurse
RMN	Registered Mental Nurse (UK)

| RNMS | Registered Nurse for Mentally Subnormal |
| SCM | State Certified Midwife |

Chiropodists (or podiatrists)

MChS	Member of the Society of Chiropodists
FChS	Fellow of the Society of Chiropodists
FCPods	Fellow of the College of Podiatrists

Appendix 2
Abbreviations commonly used within pharmacy

aa	*ana*	of each
ac	*ante cibum*	before food
ad/add	*addendus*	to be added (up to)
ad lib	*ad libitum*	as much as desired
alt	*alternus*	alternate
alt die	*alterno die*	every other day
amp	*ampulla*	ampoule
applic	*applicetur*	let it be applied
aq	*aqua*	water
aq ad	*aquam ad*	water up to
aur/aurist	*auristillae*	eardrops
bd/bid	*bis in die*	twice a day
BNF		*British National Formulary*
BP		*British Pharmacopoeia*
BPC		*British Pharmaceutical Codex*
c	*cum*	with
cap	*capsula*	capsule
cc	*cum cibus*	with food
co/comp	*compositus*	compound
collut	*collutorium*	mouthwash
conc	*concentratus*	concentrated
corp	*corpori*	to the body
crem	*cremor*	cream
d	*dies*	a day
dd	*de die*	daily
dil	*dilutus*	diluted
div	*divide*	divide
DPF		*Dental Practitioners' Formulary*
DT		*Drug Tariff*
EP		*European Pharmacopoeia*
et	*et*	and
ex aq	*ex aqua*	in water
ext	*extractum*	an extract
f/ft/fiat	*fiat*	let it be made
fort	*fortis*	strong
freq	*frequenter*	frequently
ft mist	*fiat mistura*	let a mixture be made
ft pulv	*fiat pulvis*	let a powder be made
garg	*gargarisma*	a gargle

gutt/guttae/gtt	*guttae*	drops
h	*hora*	at the hour
hs	*hora somni*	at the hour of sleep (bedtime)
ic	*inter cibos*	between meals
inf	*infusum*	infusion
inh		inhalation/inhaler
irrig	*irrigatio*	irrigation
lin	*linimentum*	liniment
liq	*liquor*	solution
lot	*lotio*	lotion
m/mane	*mane*	in the morning
md	*more dicto*	as directed
mdu	*more dicto utendus*	use as directed
mist	*mistura*	mixture
mitt/mitte	*mitte*	send (quantity to be given)
n/nocte	*nocte*	at night
n et m	*nocte maneque*	night and morning
narist	*naristillae*	nose drops
neb	*nebula*	spray
np	*nomen proprium*	the proper name
ocul	*oculo*	to (for) the eye
oculent/oc	*oculentum*	an eye ointment
od	*omni die*	every day
oh	*omni hora*	every hour
om	*omni mane*	every morning
on	*omni nocte*	every night
paa	*parti affectae applicandus*	apply to the affected part
pc	*post cibum*	after food
PC		prescriber contacted
pess	*pessus*	pessary
pig	*pigmentum*	a paint
PNC		prescriber not contacted
po	*per os*	by mouth
ppt	*praecipitatus*	precipitated
pr	*per rectum*	rectally
prn	*pro re nata*	when required
pulv	*pulvis*	a powder
pv	*per vagina*	vaginally
qds/qid	*quarter die*	four times a day
qqh/q4h	*quarta quaque hora*	every 4 hours
qs	*quantum sufficiat*	sufficient
R	*recipe*	take
rep/rept	*repetatur*	let it be repeated
sig	*signa*	let it be labelled
solv	*solve*	dissolve
sos	*si opus sit*	when necessary
stat	*statim*	immediately

supp	*suppositorium*	suppository
syr	*syrupus*	syrup
tds/tid	*ter in die*	three times a day
tinct	*tinctura*	tincture
tuss urg	*tussi urgente*	when the cough is troublesome
ung	*unguentum*	ointment
ut dict/ud	*ut dictum*	as directed
vap	*vapor*	an inhalation

Bibliography

Appelbe GE, Wingfield J (2005) *Dale and Appelbe's Pharmacy Law and Ethics*, 8th edn. London: The Pharmaceutical Press.

Baxter K, ed. (2007) *Stockley's Drug Interactions*, 8th edn. London: The Pharmaceutical Press.

British Medical Association and the Royal Pharmaceutical Society of Great Britain. *British National Formulary*, current edn. London: The Pharmaceutical Press (updated every 6 months).

British Medical Association, the Royal Pharmaceutical Society of Great Britain, the Royal College of Paediatrics and Child Health and the Neonatal and Paediatric Pharmacists Group. *British National Formulary for Children*, current edn. London: The Pharmaceutical Press (updated every year).

Department of Health (2000) *The NHS Plan*. London: The Stationery Office.

Health and Personal Social Services for Northern Ireland. *Drug Tariff*, current edn. Belfast: Central Services Agency (updated monthly).

Langley CA, Belcher D (2008) *Applied Pharmaceutical Practice*. London: The Pharmaceutical Press.

Marriot JM, Wilson KA, Langley CA, Belcher D (2006) *Pharmaceutical Compounding and Dispensing*. London: The Pharmaceutical Press.

National Health Service in Scotland. *Scottish Drug Tariff*, current edn. Edinburgh: The Scottish Executive Health Department (updated monthly online; available at: www.isdscotland.org).

National Health Service, England and Wales. *Drug Tariff*, current edn. London: The Stationery Office (updated monthly).

National Health Services Business Services Authority. Prescription Pricing Division website. Available at: www.ppa.org.uk.

Royal Pharmaceutical Society of Great Britain (2005) *The Safe and Secure Handling of Medicines: A team approach*. London: RPSGB.

Royal Pharmaceutical Society of Great Britain (2007) *Code of Ethics for Pharmacists and Pharmacy Technicians*. London: RPSGB.

Royal Pharmaceutical Society of Great Britain (2007) *Professional Standards and Guidance for the Sale and Supply of Medicines*. London: RPSGB.

Royal Pharmaceutical Society of Great Britain. *Medicines, Ethics and Practice: A guide for pharmacists and pharmacy technicians*, current edn. London: The Pharmaceutical Press (updated twice yearly).

Index